Back Pain

How to Treat Lower Back Pain with America's Foremost Expert

RONALD M LIEBERMAN, D.O.

ISBN:0615914071

ISBN-13:9780615914077

DEDICATION

This book is dedicated to my amazing children:

Jackie, Rachael, Jared and Ariel.

I would like to formally thank my publisher Randy Schrum. His incredible support and vision has made this project possible

CONTENTS

DISCLAIMER

This handbook is for informational purposes only.
It is not designed to take the place of a medical diagnoses by a competent physician.

1

HAVE YOU QUIT?

As a spine pain physician, I meet many patients who have spent years bouncing around the medical system with little to show for their efforts. Often, their previous physicians have told them that:

- "Back problems are just part of getting older."
- "You'd feel better if you lost weight."
- "According to the x-rays, you're fine."
- "Let's continue physical therapy and see what happens." (Even though nothing's happening.)
- "Here's another prescription."

Eric is one such patient. When we met, he was forty-two and had suffered from back pain for seventeen years. Despite occasional flare-ups, he led an active life that included golf, softball, skiing, and tennis. The pain was a nuisance, but he could usually manage it with ibuprofen and other over-the-counter medicines.

Six months before he visited our center, Eric's back problems worsened. At his first appointment with us, he was an 8 on a 0-10 pain scale (with 10 representing intolerable pain). His discomfort was so severe that he could no longer work or even stand long enough to shower. He'd consulted specialists at several university hospitals, including an orthopedic spine surgeon, and wasn't given much hope. The main message he'd heard was that he needed to accept the pain and "learn to live with it."

Hope for Lasting Relief

What makes messages like these so damaging is that they're flat-out wrong. I know this because I've personally worked with many hundreds of patients who came to our center discouraged, believing they were destined for a lifetime of pain and disability. Today, many of those "hopeless" cases are leading active and practically pain-free lives.

I've also worked with patients who have avoided this tugging, downward spiral of frustration and ineffective treatment. Some might call them fortunate, but often they created their own luck by studying their options and seeking out professionals who could provide appropriate care.

If you're living with chronic back pain (or have a loved one who is), this handbook was written with you in mind. In the coming chapters, we'll delve into the condition's root causes and explore the many treatments available. You'll learn to evaluate potential physicians and connect with providers who have the clinical acumen and skill to effectively diagnose and treat you. It is my sincere hope that this information will empower you to take an active role in your care so that you can find lasting relief and lead a full and active life once again.

Back Pain Hurts Everyone

If your back hurts, you're far from alone. According to the National Institute of Arthritis and Musculoskeletal and Skin Diseases, about 25 percent of Americans have at least one day of low back pain in any three-month period, and about 80 percent will deal with it at some point in their lives. Back pain is the second most common cause of disability in American adults and costs the economy over $100 billion each year in lost wages and productivity.

Studies suggest the incidence of back pain may be rising at an alarming rate. In 2006, researchers from The University of North Carolina at Chapel Hill surveyed over five thousand households to identify adults who suffered from long-term, disabling neck or back pain. When they compared their results to those of a similar survey conducted in 1992, they found that the incidence of chronic spine pain had more than doubled in just fifteen years (from 3.9 percent in 1992 to 10.2 percent in 2006). In their report, they suggested several possible causes for this trend, including rising rates of obesity and depression and patterns of increased health care seeking. However, they noted that further research is needed to delve into the trend's underlying causes.

While the triggers of back pain are complex, epidemiological research has identified several potential risk factors. Job tasks appear to play a role, as do psychosocial factors. A two-year study of over eight hundred Japanese workers identified a number of significant predictors of disabling low back pain, including a history of back problems, frequent lifting, interpersonal stress at work, and monotonous tasks. Researchers noted that these findings were consistent with those of similar studies conducted in Western countries.

Fortunately, back pain tends to be short-lived. Sixty percent of patients who see their primary care doctor due to acute (short-term) low back pain return to work within one month. However, a small minority continues to suffer from chronic, often long-term, distress. Even when it disappears quickly, back pain has a high rate of recurrence, with up to 80 percent of patients experiencing a repeat episode within a year.

Why Patients Are Frustrated

Because back pain is so common, you might assume that health care professionals know exactly how to treat it. Unfortunately, painful spinal conditions often demand complex diagnostics and management that are beyond the ability of many providers. The following are some common reasons that well-meaning physicians mismanage their patients' spine care.

Lack of Clinical Knowledge and Training

According to conventional medical wisdom, 80 to 90 percent of acute back pain cases resolve within three months— even when no treatment is provided. For this reason, most professional organizations recommend a conservative approach during this period (assuming, of course, there are no red flags of a more serious condition). Patients are usually encouraged to continue their daily activities and to control their discomfort with over-the-counter painkillers. Doctors may also prescribe physical therapy to relieve pain, strengthen the back, and improve range of motion. (We'll discuss these and other conservative treatments in detail in Chapter 3.)

Unfortunately, many health care providers are not trained to care for spine pain patients beyond the short term. So if pain doesn't go away within three months or so, they're ultimately at a loss. Dealing with chronic pain (the long-term, persistent form) is often beyond their knowledge and training. At this point, they'll often recommend ineffective, one-size-fits-all therapies and refer you to "pain management" to control your symptoms with narcotics. You may even be sent to an orthopedic surgeon for evaluation or for yet another round of physical therapy treatments.

The reality is that back pain is a highly complex condition that requires far more than the cookie-cutter management taught in many medical schools. Still, I only have to listen to my patients to know that such approaches are alive and well. One frustrated patient stated that they sometimes "feel like a pill" or only came to our specialty practice to renew their pain medication. I recently spoke to an orthopedic surgeon who says he "puts 'em on Percocet for three months, gives 'em PT [physical therapy], then sends 'em to pain management if they're not better." (Now as someone with back pain, how would such assembly line treatment make you feel?)

That being said, I believe that the vast majority of providers have high professional standards and want only the best for their patients. They simply aren't aware of the many safe and effective treatment options that might provide lasting relief. Unfortunately, they have been taught to treat the symptoms of back pain rather than delving into its root causes.

Flawed Research and Clinical Guidelines

Good physicians understand the latest medical research and incorporate it into their decision-making. Likewise, professional organizations and regulatory agencies rely on research when formulating their care recommendations. Several groups have published evidence-based clinical guidelines for low back pain care, including the International Spine Intervention Society, the American Pain Society, the American College of Physicians, and the American Society of Interventional Pain Physicians.

But as a health care provider, what do you do when the scientific evidence is contradictory, flawed, or nonexistent? This is often the case when it comes to back pain treatments. And while we've come a long way over the past decade or so, there is still a great deal of work that needs to be done.

Here's one timely example of the disconnect between research and practice. As a resident in the 1980s, I was taught that 75 percent of all acute back pain goes away on its own. (Sound familiar? As I mentioned above, this statistic is treated as conventional wisdom among many primary care providers which at one point in my career I once was, so am familiar with that milieu.) As a student, that was drilled into my head like a mantra. Based on this evidence, I was taught to reassure my back pain patients and refer them for conservative treatment (physical therapy, spinal manipulation, etc.). Only when the pain persisted beyond three months was I to recommend they see a specialist.

Sounds reasonable, right? Here's the problem. The idea that essentially all back pain, unless its cancer, an infection or fracture is self-limiting dates back to a flawed 1966 study in which British researchers examined the course of back pain by reviewing primary care physicians' appointment logs. Patients who initially sought treatment were assumed to have recovered when they stopped coming in for follow-up appointments. (Of course, the team failed to take into account the very likely scenario in which a frustrated patient changed doctors or moved on to a specialist.)

Despite its glaring flaws, this study was published in a peer-reviewed journal and became quite influential in the world of spine care. That is, until a few years ago when new evidence began emerging that suggested people with some types of back problems might be at-risk for developing chronic, degenerative spine disease. These patients, researchers warned, would likely benefit from early intervention rather than the standard wait-and-see approach. (We'll discuss early intervention further in Chapter 11).

As we delve into the scientific evidence supporting various back pain treatments, you'll notice that much of it is flawed, contradictory, or full of gaping holes. For this reason, doctors can't rely on research alone. They also need sufficient clinical judgment and experience to assess the patient's condition and decide which treatments are most promising. And as you may have noticed, finding a physician with these skills can be quite difficult.

Misled by Imaging

At some point, if your pain persists, your primary care provider will likely order imaging studies like computed tomography (CT) or magnetic resonance imaging (MRI). In many cases, this just complicates matters. While MRI is a wonderful tool for detecting fractures, tumors, infections, and herniated discs, it can't always pinpoint potentially painful spinal structures. It can also miss the true source of pain.

Case in point: When researchers in Sweden and Australia dissected the spines of people who had died in fatal car accidents, they found evidence of multiple injuries to the subjects' spinal joints, including bleeding and fractures. Interestingly, imaging studies taken before the examination had completely missed these abnormalities.

Many physicians don't understand this. When they see a "clean" film, they assume things can't be all that bad. Rather than referring you to a qualified back specialist who could diagnose and treat the root cause of your pain, they prescribe additional physical therapy or offer the old chestnut about how back pain is a normal part of aging. You may even be referred to a psychiatrist for evaluation. (In a typical workweek, I can count on meeting at least one patient who's been convinced that his or her back pain is all in the head.)

Eric: Relief at Last

Eric didn't want to "live with" chronic, debilitating pain. He was relentless about finding answers. Fortunately, he discussed the impasse with his family physician, who referred him to our center.

Understanding a patient's back pain requires quite a bit of detective work. Clues are sought and suspects eliminated. Eric's history, physical examination, imaging studies, and lab work showed no red flags of a serious underlying problem like cancer or infection. His medical workup was also negative for extraspinal problems presenting as "referred" back pain (kidney stones are a common example). This meant his pain most likely originated within his musculoskeletal system—the bones, muscles, cartilage, tendons, discs and joints that support and move the body.

At our clinic, we take a comprehensive approach to diagnosis and treatment rather than focusing on the back alone. In Eric's case, this was fortunate indeed. A head-toe-examination yielded an important clue: a tender ligament in his left foot. What's more, his heel-ankle joint was frozen to the point where I was unable to move it with my hands.

"Have you ever sprained this ankle?" I asked.

Eric laughed. "How'd you guess?"

It made perfect sense. Ankles can lock up after even a mild sprain if the patient shies away from motions that stretch the injured ligament. A healthy ankle is an excellent shock absorber that disperses considerable force with each step. But because Eric's ankle didn't move properly, it transmitted this impact upward to his spine and pelvis, causing muscle spasms and tenderness in his lower back. So ironically, the first step to treating Eric's back pain was to restore his ankle's natural mobility through a course of rehabilitation and therapeutic exercise.

Next, we needed to determine which of Eric's spinal structures actually hurt. As we'll discuss in the next chapter, the bones of the spine are connected by a series of joints that allow our backs to twist and bend. Even relatively young people can develop arthritis in one or more of these spinal joints. On imaging studies, several of Eric's joints showed signs of wear and tear. His history—nagging back pain that gradually worsened over a period of years—also suggested joint involvement.

So which of Eric's joints was the culprit? We couldn't rely on imaging alone, because not all degenerative joint changes are actually painful. To pinpoint the problem, we used x-ray-guidance to inject a small volume of local anesthetic onto the spinal nerve branches to the spinal column joints on the painful side of Eric's back. These are the same nerves that carry sensory signals from the spinal joints to the brain. Once he was numb, we had him twist in ways that had previously aggravated his back—and found he was completely pain free. We repeated the procedure a few days later to rule out a placebo response (in other words, an improvement not due to the injection). The second dose of anesthetic also relieved his pain, which suggested his joints were indeed the problem.

After we'd confidently identified the root cause of Eric's problem, I treated him with a minimally invasive procedure called radiofrequency ablation. This involves inserting a needle probe along the course of the spinal nerve branches we'd previously numbed. The probe emits radio signals that create heat, which cauterizes the nerves and interrupts that transmission of pain signals. Like many patients, Eric experienced some mild side effects afterward, including muscle spasms, which disappeared within a week.

Eric's response was excellent. For the first time in seventeen years, his back was pain free. He returned to work and was soon playing golf and tennis several times a week. Today, he takes no pain medications and sees me only once a year for follow-up treatment.

Where I'm Coming From

Every nonfiction author brings their unique experiences, education, and beliefs to their material. Since I've encouraged you to vet your doctors' backgrounds, I suppose it's only fair that I share my own before we go further.

Long before I settled on medicine as a career, I aspired to be a professional musician. Even after I switched gears and enrolled in medical school, I continued to study the trumpet with the best teachers I could find. Forty years later, I've finally reached the level where I can play semiprofessionally with a contemporary big band outfit (though I'm not about to quit my day job).

Trumpet skills may not seem like an impressive credential for a spine pain specialist, but the two disciplines have more in common than meets the eye. If you've ever worked on mastering an instrument, you know that it requires diligence, patience, and follow through. It taught me certain habits of mind—focus, patience, and above all persistence—that have served me well as a spine pain specialist.

Like many physicians, I chose a career in medicine out of a genuine desire to relieve others' suffering. I completed my internship at the (now-defunct) Metropolitan Hospital in Philadelphia, caring for extremely sick patients with multi-system illnesses. Afterward, I was contemplating a number of career directions when, out of the blue, I was offered a residency in physical medicine and rehabilitation.

I had a chance encounter during my residency experience that led me to a physician who was treating back pain through a combination of therapeutic exercise and x-ray-guided spinal injections. I was intrigued by the excellent outcomes this doctor was achieving and excited to find an approach that directly addressed the root causes of back pain.

The technique I witnessed was an example of interventional Physical Medicine and Rehabilitation (Physiatry) that focuses on minimally invasive treatments in the context of therapeutic exercising. Back in the mid-1990s, the field had just begun to take off. There were only about four unofficial fellowships available in the entire country, and all had yearlong waiting lists. But if I'd learned anything from my music studies, it was the importance of studying under the best. When one of the top minds in the field lectured in my area, I made sure to attend and introduce myself. A year later, I loaded a suitcase with books and journal articles and headed to New Orleans for a four-day crash course with a physician considered to be one of the gurus of interventional spine pain diagnostics.

I can't tell you how eye-opening that experience was. I witnessed techniques to locate and verify the true source of pain and studied unnerving cases in which surgeons "operated on images" rather than delving deeper into the underlying pathology. The importance of creativity, problem solving, and listening was emphasized. After long days of lecturing, the instructor sat with me into the night, generously answering a year's worth of my accumulated questions.

The experience changed the course of my life. Many years, classes, and fellowship experiences later, I now practice interventional physical medicine in a way that is both intellectually challenging and spiritually satisfying, offering treatments that make a huge difference in patient lives. I'm proud and humbled when someone says, "No one's ever examined me like this before!" or "I've never had so much insight into all the possibilities!" I have also been privileged to pass on my knowledge as a teaching faculty member at conferences of the North American Spine Society and International Spine Intervention Society. I look forward to the day when clinical knowledge of back pain is equal across the board amongst all physicians, and when all patients are believed, understood, and promptly referred to the appropriate level of care.

Next Steps

If you're in pain—and you really want help—don't let your doctor tell you "your x-rays are normal" or "it's just part of getting old." Don't settle for "it's all in your head" or "just deal with it." Take charge of your care by learning everything you can about the science and treatment of back pain and connecting with a provider who can help you. May this book serve as your road map on the path to relief and recovery.

2

WHAT HAS ANATOMY GOT TO DO WITH IT?

If your back hurts, you may wonder how you got yourself into this mess in the first place. Was it the time you threw your toddler into the air, only to find she'd gained a few pounds since her previous launch? Or are your years of varsity rowing in high school and college catching up with you? Maybe you're doing too much heavy lifting at work or spending too much time in front of a computer.

The answer could be all of these—or none of them. Research suggests that back pain arises from a complex interplay of genes, environment, and body mechanics. To understand how things go wrong, it's helpful to know how the many structures of your back function and interact. So before we dive any deeper into individual conditions and treatments, let's take a closer look at the spine itself.

Spinal Anatomy 101

To help you through your daily activities, the bones, nerves, discs, ligaments, and muscles of your back must work seamlessly together. A disturbance in any one of these components can affect the others. An irritated spinal joint, for example, might cause painful spasms in the nearby muscles.

The following is a roster of the key lower back "players" and their functions:

Bones

Your spinal column consists of a stack of smallish bones called vertebral bodies that descends from the base of your skull to your pelvis. It's held together by a series of strong ligaments, pads of fibrous tissue called intervertebral discs, and a series of joints called the zygopophyseal or z-joints.

The lower spine is divided into three regions, or curves:

- The **lumbar (lower back) curve** includes the five largest vertebrae, which are called L1 to S1 in descending order. It extends from your waist to your pelvis. This region supports your upper-body weight and makes it possible for you to bend, twist at the hips, and lift heavy objects.

- The **sacral (pelvic) curve** consists of five fused vertebrae that rest in the pelvic cavity and attach to the ilium, or hipbone, on either side. These junctures, known as the sacraliliac (SI) joints, support the weight of the entire spinal column. The sacral bones are named S1 through S5, again in descending order.

- The **coccygeal (tailbone) curve** forms lowest portion of the spine, or coccyx. It consists of three to five rudimentary vertebrae that may or may not be fused. Commonly called the tailbone, it serves as an important attachment point for muscles and ligaments.

Your spinal column's most important job is to protect the spinal cord and nerve roots that transmit signals between your brain and lower body. All vertebrae (except the very lowest) consist of a cylindrical body with several spines, or processes, that enclose and protect these delicate structures.

In addition, the spine supports your upper body and allows you to bend and move. It also serves as an attachment point for the muscles of your torso, notably the erector spinae muscles of the back.

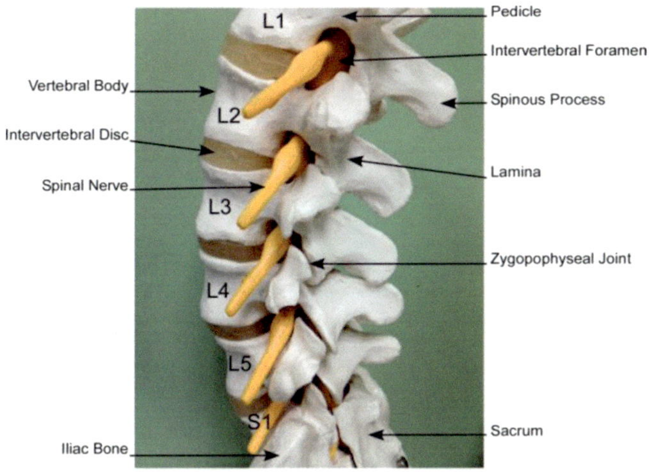

Figure 1: Basic lumbar spine anatomy. Note the presence of the intervertebral foramen boundaries to pedicles on the top and bottom, discs in the front, and joints and lamina in the back.

Discs

The intervertebral discs are flat bands of fibrous cartilage that lie between the main bodies of the lumbar vertebrae. Each consists of a tough outer layer (the annulus fibrosus) and a gel-like inner layer (the nucleus pulposus). The discs are attached to the vertebrae on either side by tough cartilage end plates.

Collectively, the discs cushion the vertebrae and serve as torque converters that distribute force up and down the spinal column. They also act as ligaments that attach one vertebra to the next while allowing for slight movement.

The intervertebral discs are among the largest organs in the body that don't have a direct blood supply. In a healthy disc, only the outer third of the annulus is supplied by blood vessels. Within the nucleus, nutrients and waste products must be transported by diffusion. This works best when the nucleus is evenly pressurized, well hydrated, and rich in water-binding proteins called proteoglycans.

Likewise, in a healthy disc, only the outer part of the annulus is innervated, (or in other words, wired with sensory nerve endings). In theory, this means that only the surface of the annulus can feel pain.

However, wear and tear to the disc surface sometimes allows nerve endings to invade deeper into the disc where they can become sensitive and irritated. This "neoinnervation" is believed to be an important contributing factor in some cases of back pain.

Z-Joints

Flexion and twisting of the back is guided by a series of joints in the rear portion of the spine known as zygapophyseal or z-joints. These are formed where the spinous processes of adjacent vertebrae meet. Each is enclosed in a capsule, which includes a fibrous outer "envelope" rich in nerve endings. The inner capsule is filled with synovial fluid, a kind of natural lubricant that reduces bone-on-bone friction during movement (similar to the fluid that bathes larger joints like your knees).

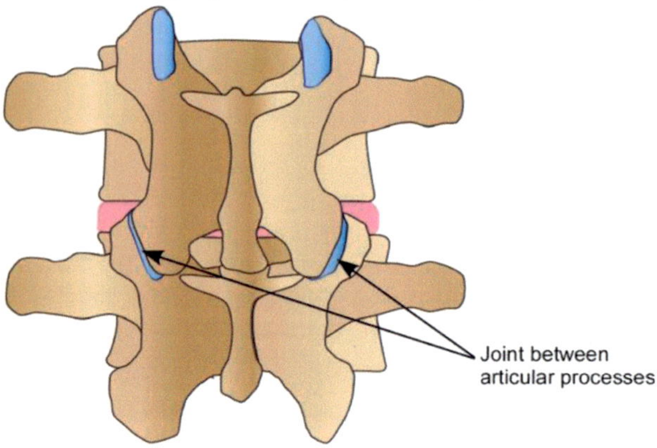

Figure 2: Note the cartilage covering of the z-joints

The z-joints are innervated by the medial branch nerves, which derive from the spinal nerves at the same level. In addition to transmitting sensory info, the medial branch nerve controls movement of small muscles called the multifidi that lie deep in the back and are believed to assist in coordinating and stabilizing spine movement.

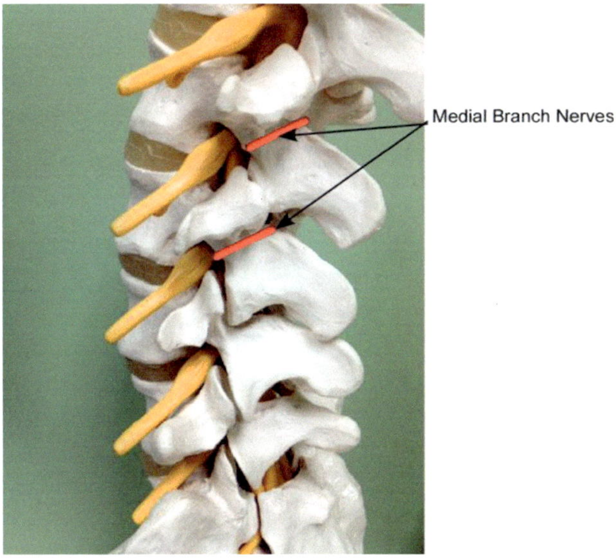

Figure 3: Typical location of medial branch nerves. The sensory portion of these nerves allow the z-joints to feel pain.

Sacroiliac (SI) Joints

The two SI joints lie at the juncture of the ilium (hipbone) and the sacrum (which forms the pelvic portion of the spine) and are held together by a series of strong ligaments. Like the z-joints, they are contained within nerve-rich capsules.

A healthy SI joint is extremely stable. The convex surface of the ileum and concave surface of the sacrum are designed to lock together under pressure. Movement in either SI joint produces reflected movement in its counterpart.

The nerve structure of the SI joints differs somewhat from person to person. Each joint receives innervation from both the lateral branch nerves and sacral nerves as well as the dorsal rami of the L5 spinal nerve. Different nerves enter the joint from different directions to create a complex neural network.

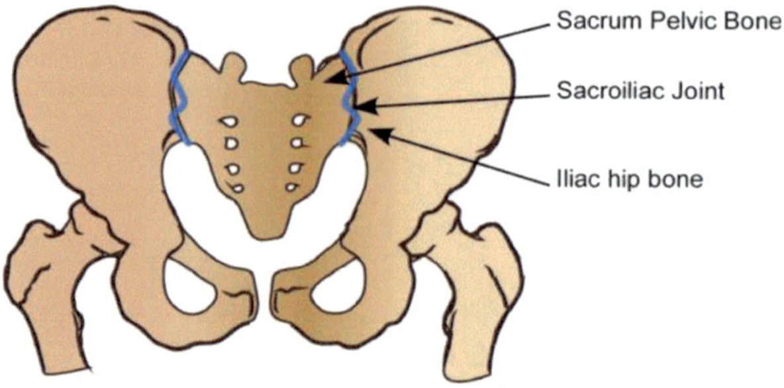

Figure 4: This is a schematic cartoon of the sacroiliac joint and its "S" shaped configuration. Like the z-joint, it is lined with cartilage.

Spinal Nerves

The spinal cord is a rope-like bundle of nerve tissue that extends from the base of the brainstem to the upper lumbar spine. These delicate structures are protected against trauma by the boney spinal canal, which is formed by the vertebral bodies, spinous processes, and facet joints. A thin covering of bone called the lamina lies along the length of this canal on either side of the spinous processes.

The spinal cord acts as the switchboard of the back, transmitting nerve signals between the brain and much of the body. It can even control some movements and processes independently. For example, if you accidentally touch a hot pan, your spinal cord triggers a reflex that causes you to jerk your hand away. Reflexes are also believed to play a role in the locking of your SI joints under extreme loading.

The spinal cord is divided into thirty-one segments. At each level, pairs of nerve "rootlets" branch out from both sides. Rootlets join to form roots, and roots coalesce into larger nerves that exit the boney spinal column through openings known as neuroforamina (or simply foramina). Each set of spinal nerves transmits motor and sensory signals to part of the lower body.

The area of skin innervated by a certain spinal nerve is called a dermatome. For example, the spinal nerves originating at L5 transmit sensory signals to a band of skin that runs the entire length of the leg. In some cases, pain or sensory changes within a dermatome can provide important clues about the cause of your back pain.

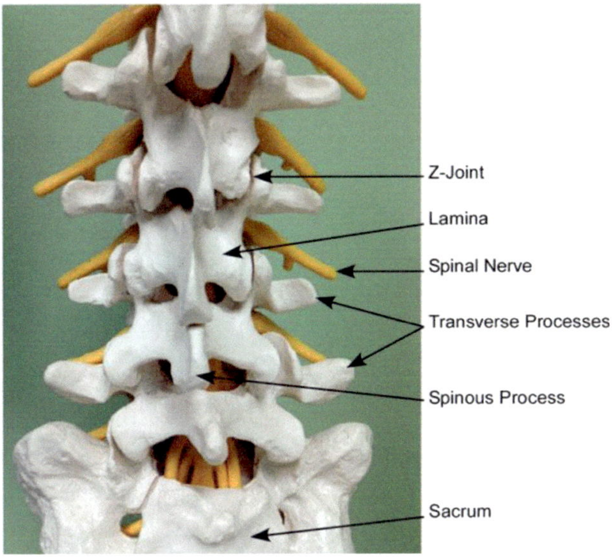

Figure 5: Viewing the spine from behind on the posterior side. The spinal nerve is depicted coming out from underneath of the roof or lamina. The z-joints share the posterior lateral (side) wall of the spine. The transverse and spinous processes are some of the muscular attachment sites that both restrain and guide spine motion.

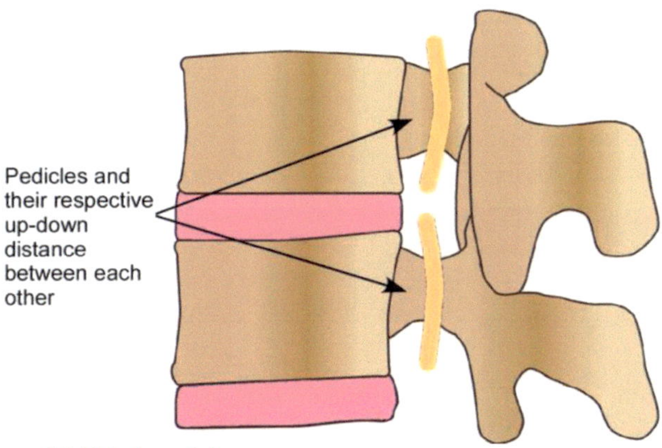

Figure 6: Lateral (side) view of the nerves.

The Physiology of Pain

Unfortunately, we all know what pain feels like. But what really causes that burning, tingling, aching, and throbbing that drive you crazy and keep you awake at night?

The answer is complex and depends on the body structures and chemical processes involved. For our purposes, back pain comes in three varieties: nociceptive, neuropathic, and mixed.

Nociceptive Pain

Nociceptive pain occurs when sensory nerve endings (called nociceptors) detect temperature, pressure, or chemical changes (bleach burning your skin, for example). Nociceptive pain is usually structural in origin—in other words, it signals that some body tissue has been physically damaged. Examples include sprains, bruises, fractures, and arthritis.

Nociceptors are found practically everywhere in the body, including the spine. When triggered to a certain threshold (the potato is too hot, that slap was too hard), they release a rush of pain-transmitting chemicals, including a sensory neuropeptide called Substance P. These set off a chain reaction of events that transmit distress signals to your central nervous system, which are experienced by you as pain.

The release of pain chemicals also activates an inflammatory response around the affected nerve, which is designed to purge harmful stimuli and promote tissue healing. However, prolonged inflammation can increase your nerves' sensitivity to pain. Left untreated, chronic inflammation can also damage and degrade certain tissues, leading to even more pain and disability.

Neuropathic (nerve) Pain

This pain type occurs when the nerves themselves are irritated or compressed. People often describe it as sharp, stabbing, burning, or tingly. It's sometimes accompanied by signs of nerve dysfunction (neuropathy) such as sensory changes, muscle weakness, or diminished reflexes in the legs.

Possible causes of spinal nerve pain include:

- **Herniated intervertebral disc.** A bulge or bump in the disc presses on a nerve.
- **Chemical irritation.** The nucleus pulposus is made of nerve-irritating material that can protrude through tears in the annulus and inflame nearby nerve tissue.
- **Spinal stenosis.** Narrowing of the spinal canal due to structural degeneration and subsequent nerve irritation. The pain is often aggravated by particular movements.
- **Foreign bodies.** Examples include dislodged medical devices and fluid that accumulates due to injury or infection.
- **Cancer.** Tumors can compress the spinal cord and nerve roots.
- **Shingles.** In people who have had the chicken pox, the virus can flare up and attack the spinal nerves.
- **Vitamin deficiencies.**
- **Medications, including some kinds of chemotherapy.**
- **Nerve damage due to diabetes.**

Though neuropathic pain can be intense and debilitating, it doesn't necessarily signal physical damage to the nerve. For a variety of reasons we'll explore later, nerves sometimes malfunction and send out pain signals when no actual tissue damage has occurred.

Compared to the nociceptive type, nerve pain tends to last longer and can be more difficult to treat. However, recent advances have made it possible for most patients to find significant relief and improve their quality of life.

Mixed-Category Pain

It's possible for a single condition to cause both pain types. Disc herniation, for example, can cause nocioceptive back pain (originating in the disc itself) and neuropathic leg pain (due to irritation of the associated spinal nerve). Both must be treated to provide maximum relief.

Types of Back Pain

When you see a doctor about low back pain, what should you expect? Your visit will usually begin with a thorough medical history and physical exam. This involves examining your back by touch and observing you as you stand, walk, bend, twist, and squat. Your doctor may also test your reflexes and probe for possible neurological issues by checking strength and sensation in your feet and legs. If your pain radiates into your lower extremities, you may be asked to raise each leg slowly while lying on your back or sitting. This movement increases stress on your spinal nerve roots and can provide important clues about the origins of your pain.

After examining you, your doctor will generally take one of three approaches, depending on the exam findings.

Underlying Medical Conditions

On rare occasions, low back pain can signal a dangerous underlying problem such as a tumor or organ dysfunction. Red flags of a potentially serious condition include:

- **A history of recent trauma**
- **Fever**
- **Bowel or bladder incontinence**
- **Unexplained weight loss**
- **A history of cancer**
- **Long-term steroid use**
- **Intravenous drug abuse**
- **Intense, localized pain**
- **Limited range of motion**
- **Inability to get into a comfortable position**

If your doctor suspects that your back pain is due to an underlying condition, he or she will generally order a thorough workup, including imaging studies and laboratory tests. Medical conditions that sometimes cause back pain are described in the next section.

Radicular Low Back Pain (Sciatica)

Sciatica is back pain that radiates into your lower extremities. It's sometimes accompanied by numbness, tingling, or weakness of the legs. Radiating pain usually indicates compression or irritation of the spinal nerve roots.

Simple Low Back Pain

Non-radicular back pain is usually caused by mechanical problems of the muscles, bones, ligaments, discs, or joints. Though it's most often concentrated in the low back, it can also cause discomfort in the buttocks, groin, or upper legs.

Medical Conditions That Cause Back Pain

Sometimes back pain can be a sign of an underlying medical problem. This might originate within the spine itself or elsewhere in the lower abdomen. Some disorders of the urinary, digestive, and cardiovascular systems can actually send pain to the low back region. This phenomenon is known as "referred pain," and it can be quite difficult to distinguish from true spine pain.

Kidney Stones (Nephrolithiasis)

Minerals in urine sometimes solidify or crystallize in the kidneys. If the resulting stone grows too large (three millimeters or bigger), it can lodge in the channels of the kidney or ureter, resulting in severe pain on one side of the body. The discomfort often comes in waves and may radiate toward the groin or genitals. You may also notice blood or pus in your urine or pain during urination. The condition is most common in men.

In many cases, patients can be treated with painkillers until the stone passes naturally. Certain medications and non-invasive ultrasonic energy treatments can break up larger stones. Surgery is sometimes required.

Cancer and Tumors

Benign and malignant tumors can invade the spine, causing simple or radicular back pain. Cancer may originate in the spine itself (often as bone cancer) or spread from elsewhere in the body. Multiple myeloma, a type of blood cancer, often causes painful bone lesions on the vertebrae. In addition to back pain, the person may notice unexplained fever or weight loss.

If you have both back pain and a history of cancer, it's important to get a thorough workup, including laboratory tests and imaging studies. Once properly diagnosed, cancer and other tumors can be treated with a combination of surgery, chemotherapy, and radiation therapy.

Infectious Diseases

Many bacteria and viruses have been known to attack the vertebrae and spinal cord. Tuberculosis, for example, may spread to the spine from the lungs. Even the flu can cause spine complications in rare cases.

Spine infections are particularly common in people with a history of intravenous drug abuse and those with weakened immune systems. Back pain due to infection is often accompanied by fever. Once properly diagnosed, the condition can be treated with appropriate medications, including antibiotics or antiviral drugs.

Hyperparathyroidism

Overactivity of the parathyroid glands (small glands located on the thyroid gland itself) has many causes, including endocrine dysfunction, tumors, vitamin D deficiency, and kidney disease.

Parathyroid hormone regulates blood levels of calcium and phosphate, two minerals essential to bone health. Too much calcium in the bloodstream can cause muscle and bone pain, including low back pain. Patients may also notice symptoms like constipation, kidney stones, nausea, and vomiting.

Certain laboratory tests can detect excess parathyroid hormone in the blood. Treatment usually involves resolving any underlying causes as well as medication therapy to regulate blood calcium levels.

Abdominal Aortic Aneurysm (AAA)

The aorta, the body's largest artery, extends downward from the heart through the abdomen, supplying the lower body with oxygen-rich blood. In rare cases, the abdominal portion of the vessel balloons or bulges. This distended area sometimes extends to the iliac arteries of the pelvis.

AAA usually has no symptoms, but may present as pulsing pain in the chest, abdomen, scrotum, or lower back. It's most common in men ages sixty-five to seventy-five who have a history of cigarette smoking. Due to the risk of rupture, painful cases are often treated surgically.

Lupus Disease

Systemic lupus erythematosus is a chronic, incurable autoimmune disease in which the body's own immune system attacks healthy tissue. Lupus tends to occur in flares and may cause periods of fever, skin problems, and joint pain (including back pain). Lab tests can detect certain antibodies characteristic of the disease. Treatment includes painkillers and medications to reduce the frequency of flares.

Shingles

Shingles (herpes zoster) is a viral disease caused by the chickenpox (varicella zoster) virus. After the initial infection (usually in childhood), the virus lies latent in the nerve roots of the spinal cord. It can flare up years or even decades later, resulting in intensely painful skin blisters. In rare cases, pain radiates along a single spinal nerve, but causes no rash on the associated skin surface.

Shingles can cause rare but serious neurological complications, including inflammation of the spinal cord. Laboratory tests are needed to detect disease-specific antigens in the blood. Antiviral and steroid drugs can shorten the illness and relieve pain.

Vitamin Deficiencies

When adults don't get enough vitamin D or calcium, their bones gradually become less mineral-dense. This may lead to pain, muscle weakness, and fractures (often after very mild trauma such as stepping or sitting down). Over time, untreated vitamin deficiencies can lead to loss of height and skeletal deformity.

Routine bone density and blood testing can detect deficiencies early and prevent trouble down the road. Dietary supplements and weight bearing exercise can help to stabilize the condition and promote bone health.

Scientific Research: How Do We Know?

Throughout this book, we'll be discussing the latest research on common back pain treatments. If you're new to experimental design and reporting, here's a quick primer on the process. As an example, we'll follow the trials of an imaginary painkiller called Wondrex.

To test the effects of Wondrex on low back pain, researchers begin by designing an experiment. This needs to be done carefully, because the results won't be meaningful if their methods are flawed. They decide to conduct a controlled trial, which compares patients treated with Wondrex against a control group who receives no treatment. This allows them to draw strong conclusions about the drug's effectiveness. (Without the control group, they won't know whether improvement is due to the drug or the patients simply got better over time.)

Ideally, the participants won't know which group they're in. To ensure this, the team gives the control group a placebo—a "sham" or "fake" treatment that looks like Wondrex but has no real effect. This ensures that psychological factors don't influence the study results.

As the experiment proceeds, the researchers visit with patients to measure their response to treatment. Because this is a low back pain study, participants are asked to rate their pain intensity on a scale of 0-10 and fill out a standardized questionnaire that measures their functional ability (ability to perform routine life tasks). They're also asked to report any side effects they've experienced.

Once the experiment concludes, the scientists use statistical analysis to measure the outcome differences between the Wondrex and control groups. Did the participants who took Wondrex improve more than those who took the placebo? Differences that can't be accounted for by chance are said to be statistically significant. Ideally, these results are then published in peer-reviewed journals or presented at scientific conferences so researchers, clinicians, and patients can benefit.

Once a number of Wondrex trials are published, researchers can perform a systematic review (also called a meta-analysis). By combining and analyzing outcome data across several studies, they can form stronger conclusions about Wondrex's risks and benefits. One important source for reviews is the Cochrane Collaboration, a respected global network of researchers that conducts and updates analyses on key health care topics.

As you'll see in coming chapters, not all back pain treatments are well studied. Lack of research doesn't necessarily mean an approach is ineffective. However, when evidence for a treatment is limited, your physician will need to rely on experience and clinical judgment. This is another reason why it's important to work with the most experienced back pain specialist available.

Key Points

- For your spine to function properly, your bones, discs, joints, muscles, and ligaments must all work together. A problem in any of these structures can affect the others.

- Pain comes in different types. Nociceptive pain is caused by tissue damage, while nerve pain results when a nerve is compressed or irritated. Both are common in people with back pain, and they can even occur together.

- Back pain may be confined to the back itself or radiate into the lower body. The latter type is called sciatica or radicular pain.

- Back pain can sometimes be an emergency, especially when it's caused by a serious underlying condition. See your doctor immediately if your pain is severe or accompanied by other "red flag" symptoms.

Now that you're familiar with medical research, let's see what the evidence says about some common treatments. We'll begin with conservative care—gentle, noninvasive interventions that are commonly prescribed as first-line therapy for low back pain..

3

THE BENEFITS AND PITFALLS OF CONSERVATIVE TREATMENT

When Mr. Jones, age forty-eight, felt a twinge of pain in his lower back while putting up the Christmas tree, he wasn't worried. After he'd aggravated his back a few years ago, he'd rested in bed for two days, taken a few Advil, and ended up good as new. So he put his teenage sons in charge of tree duty while he relaxed on the couch.

Over the next few days, the pain got worse. Soon it was so intense he could barely concentrate at work, and sometimes it kept him up at night. After suffering for two weeks, he finally made an appointment to see his family physician.

Dr. Keen reassured him that he had no "red flags" that might indicate a serious problem. In all likelihood, it was just a sprain that would heal on its own. She prescribed stronger anti-inflammatories, muscle relaxants, and physical therapy.

At their twice-a-week sessions, the therapist treated Mr. Jones with ultrasound and hot compresses. She gave him an electrotherapy unit to use at home and recommended weekly massages. He followed all of her suggestions, but the pain persisted.

When Mr. Jones arrived at his follow-up appointment clutching the right side of his back, Dr. Keen ordered an MRI. The radiologist's report noted signs of degenerative disc disease and nonspecific spondylosis (spinal arthritis). Dr. Keen recommended a chiropractor, and Mr. Jones, who was growing more and more distressed, agreed to go (even though his insurance wouldn't cover the treatments). At first, spinal manipulation helped, but within two months his pain had returned.

"I guess it's time to consult an orthopedic surgeon," Dr. Keen said at his follow-up appointment.

Mr. Jones was surprised. "Why? I don't have any fractures." But by this point, he was willing to try anything.

The surgeon didn't think Mr. Jones needed an operation, but he did recommend yet another therapist who was getting great results for people with back pain. Reluctantly, Mr. Jones agreed to try physical therapy again. On the way home, he filled prescriptions for Percocet and another muscle relaxant.

Once again, Mr. Jones gave his all in therapy, but it didn't relieve his pain. When he voiced his frustration, the therapist suggested he try acupuncture. That seemed to help—he walked out of his session feeling great for the first time in months. But the next day, the pain returned.

Mr. Jones was at the end of his rope. He hadn't slept well in months, hadn't thrown the football with his son, and his work performance was suffering. His wife had been supportive at first, but now her jokes about their non-existent sex life were starting to sound like threats.

"Why can't anyone help me?" he complained to Dr. Keen at his next appointment. "I can't keep going like this."

"You seem down," said Dr. Keen. "I've got the name of a great psychiatrist..."

Too Much of a Good Thing?

If Mr. Jones' experience sounds familiar, rest assured you're not alone. At our center, we see many people who have been through months, years, and even decades of ineffective conservative treatment. Often, they're convinced that no one can help them, or that their doctors don't believe them, or even that they're going crazy. They've never heard about the many interventional and surgical treatments that have a good record for treating back pain.

Conservative care can be a good strategy during the acute stage of back pain. While new research is debunking the idea that most spine pain is self-limiting, many people do recover within a few weeks—even if their provider does nothing more than reassure them. This is especially true in cases involving strains and sprains, which tend to heal quickly and completely.

The trouble usually starts when the problem persists beyond three months. At this point, many providers continue to treat their patients conservatively—even when this approach is not supported by research. Often they'll prescribe more physical therapy and stronger medications and then refer the person to "pain management." Too often, this means indiscriminate treatment with narcotics. (Believe it or not, I occasionally see back pain patients who have been prescribed Percocet on an "as needed" basis.) Many patients are also referred for surgical consultation, though relatively few go on to have operations. The rest get stuck in conservative care limbo for months—or even years.

Even when conscientious primary care providers take time to delve into the latest research or consult colleagues, they don't always receive clear guidance. As noted in the clinical guidelines of the American College of Physicians (ACP), "There has been little consensus, either within or between specialties, on appropriate clinical evaluation and management of low back pain. Numerous studies show unexplained, large variations in use of diagnostic tests and treatments."

This is where educating yourself and becoming an expert in your own condition can really make a difference. By understanding the benefits and limitations of conservative treatment, you'll be able to play a more active role in your care—and recognize when it's time to move on to more aggressive treatments.

Conservative Care: What the Research Says

The remainder of this chapter examines the scientific evidence behind the most popular conservative treatments. (For additional information on how to evaluate medical research, see Chapter 3.)

One caveat before we begin: scientific evidence is a valuable tool that can inform physicians' decision-making. However, just because the benefits of a certain treatment aren't borne out by research doesn't make it useless or wrong. Trials of spinal manipulation have not shown many long-term benefits for people with chronic low back pain. However, I personally see a chiropractor every now and then because I am helped. In addition, I've referred many people for physical therapy and therapeutic exercise because I know from my years of clinical experience which patients are likely to benefit.

The same is true of more aggressive treatments. As we'll see in Chapter

9, spine surgery has received a bad rap. In my opinion, this is because too many surgeons "operate on images" without ordering a thorough diagnostic workup or considering psychosocial issues like depression. Fortunately, I am blessed to have worked with talented surgeons who achieve excellent outcomes because they consider the big picture when making decisions.

Bottom line: the best treatment decisions are based on both the scientific evidence and your doctor's clinical judgment and experience. With that in mind, let's see what the research says about the treatments Mr. Jones received.

Bed Rest

Occasionally, you'll find a primary care provider who still recommends a week or longer of bed rest for low back pain. It's true that lying down often relieves the discomfort by taking pressure off the spinal muscles, joints, and discs. However, relaxing in bed for long periods probably won't help you heal any faster—and could make things worse.

In 2005, the Cochrane Collaboration Back Review Group carried out a systematic review of four high-quality studies involving nearly nine hundred patients. The results suggested that staying active had a positive effect that was "small but consistent" in patients with acute low back pain. Conversely, patients who rested in bed for at least two days reported slightly more pain and disability and had missed more days of work at both four and twelve weeks follow-up.

Based on these findings, the ACP recommends that patients with acute back pain avoid prolonged bed rest. Try to maintain your daily routine as much as possible, even if you need to lie down briefly. Judicious use of appropriate medications may help you to maintain a higher activity level, which will promote faster healing.

It's worth noting that not all patients benefit from staying active. The Cochrane team found that study participants with sciatica had the same amount of pain and disability at follow-up whether they stayed in bed or not.

Medications

If your pain is severe or keeping you from your daily activities, your physician will likely recommend medication. A wide variety of drugs have demonstrated short-term benefits for people with low back pain. However, because the long-term risks of many medications are not well-studied, drugs should be viewed as a temporary measure that can provide relief until your body heals itself or the underlying problem is treated.

Here's what we know about the safety and efficacy of the most commonly prescribed back pain medications.

Mild Analgesics

Examples: acetaminophen (Tylenol)

The ACP recommends mild painkillers such as acetaminophen and NSAIDs (discussed below) as first-line treatments for low back pain. Acetaminophen is inexpensive and widely available without a prescription. When taken as recommended, it's safe for most people. However, it can be toxic in high doses and in patients with certain medical conditions (notably liver disease and alcoholism).

Non-steroidal Anti-inflammatory Drugs (NSAIDs)

Examples: ibuprofen (Advil, Motrin, Nuprin); naproxen (Aleve); celecoxib (Celebrex); ketoprofen (Actron, Orudis KT)

NSAIDs inhibit the production of certain enzymes that cause pain and inflammation. They are among the most frequently prescribed drugs worldwide. Some are available over the counter, while others require a prescription.

In 2008, the Cochrane Collaboration conducted a thorough systematic review of NSAID therapy for low back pain. Their analysis included sixty-five randomized, controlled trials involving over eleven thousand patients. Results suggested that NSAIDS provided modest short-term relief for both acute and chronic low back pain. All NSAIDs studied had similar effect sizes. However, the team found moderate evidence that NSAIDs were no better at relieving low back pain than acetaminophen, which had a better safety profile.

A major drawback of NSAIDs is the risk of adverse effects, including stomach ulcers, stomach bleeding, heart attack, stroke, high blood pressure, and kidney damage. Results of the Cochrane Review suggested that a newer class of NSAIDs called COX-2 inhibitors caused significantly fewer adverse effects than traditional NSAIDs. However, the team qualified these findings by pointing to a possible link between COX-2 inhibitors and serious cardiac events.

The ACP advises physicians to take a conservative approach when recommending NSAIDs. Ideally, patients should take the lowest effective dose for the shortest period possible. Therefore, it's wise to discuss alternative medications with your physician if your pain is severe or lasts more than a few weeks.

Muscle Relaxants

Examples: cyclobenzaprine (Flexeril); carisoprodol (Soma); tizanidine (Zanaflex); chlorzoxazone (Parafon Forte); metaxalone (Skelaxin); methocarbamol (Robaxin); orphenadrine (Norflex)

Muscle relaxants are a diverse group of medications used to treat musculoskeletal problems and spasticity. They are frequently prescribed for low back pain, often in conjunction with NSAIDs.

The use of muscle relaxant therapy in the treatment of back pain is controversial. A 2003 systematic review by van Tulder and colleagues found that muscle relaxants were generally effective in providing short-term relief for patients with both acute and chronic low back pain. However, they were also likely to cause adverse effects, especially severe drowsiness. Other common side effects included headache, blurred vision, nausea, vomiting, and a small risk of dependency.

Van Tulder's team concluded that muscle relaxants should be prescribed with caution and that additional trials are needed to determine whether they are in fact more effective than mild analgesics and NSAIDs. These recommendations are echoed by the ACP guidelines, which urge physicians to weigh the risk of adverse effects against potential benefits when prescribing these medications.

Opioid analgesics

Examples: hydrocodone (Vicodin); codeine (Tylenol with Codeine); oxycodone (Percocet, Oxycontin); hydromorphone (Palladone, Dilaudid); tramadol (Rybix, Ryzolt, Ultram)

Opioid analgesics are among the most potent painkillers available and have been used to relieve human suffering since before recorded history.

They are often prescribed for patients who are in severe pain due to surgery, trauma, or cancer. Due to their popularity with recreational users and potential for abuse, many opioids are classified as narcotics and controlled substances.

A 2004 systematic review by Kalso and colleagues found that opioids were quite effective in relieving both musculoskeletal and nerve-induced back pain, with most studies reporting at least a 30 percent decrease in participants' average pain intensity. However, because opioids are physically and psychologically addictive, their use in the treatment of back pain remains controversial.

For one thing, there's little evidence that opioids, particularly weaker ones, are more effective than safer, less addictive drugs. A 2006 analysis by Furlan and colleagues examined eight high-quality trials that compared the effects of opioids to those of NSAIDs and tricyclic antidepressants. They found that while strong opioids (oxycodone, morphine) were significantly more effective at relieving chronic pain, weaker ones (codeine, tramadol) did not demonstrate any notable advantages over other pain medications.

The relationship between back pain and substance abuse is not well-studied. However, results of a 2007 systematic review conducted at the Yale University School of Medicine found that as many as 43 percent of patients participating in opioid trials met the clinical criteria for substance abuse disorder, and between 5 and 24 percent disobeyed the dosage instructions of their physician or pharmacist.

The high incidence of adverse effects is yet another potential drawback of opioid therapy. The Kalso review found that 80 percent of opioid trial participants experienced at least one side effect such as constipation, nausea, or sleepiness. These problems are far less common in patients treated with NSAIDs and tricyclic antidepressants.

In summary, opioid therapy can have both significant benefits and significant risks. The ACP recommends its conservative, short-term use for patients who are suffering from severe or disabling back pain that doesn't respond to other types of medication. Physicians are urged to carefully weigh potential risks and benefits before recommending opioid therapy.

Antiepileptics

Examples: gabapentin (Neurontin); pregabalin (Lyrica)

Preliminary studies suggest that certain anti-seizure medications provide modest, short-term relief in people with sciatica. A 2001 clinical trial involving sixty-five subjects found that a six-week course of gabapentin-therapy relieved both radiating and movement-induced leg pain (though it had minimal effect on back pain). A second trial carried out two years later with fifty patients found that an eight-week course of gabapentin therapy significantly reduced patients' pain at rest while improving their motor function, sensory function, and range of motion.

While these results are promising, the FDA has not yet approved anti-seizure medication for the treatment of back pain. Further studies are needed to explore the effectiveness of this approach and compare its risks and benefits to those of other painkillers.

Tricyclic Antidepressants

Examples: amitriptyline (Elavil); nortriptyline (Pamelor); desipramine (Norpramin); doxepin (Silenor, Zonalon); imipramine (Tofranil)

Emerging evidence suggests that depression and pain share common biological pathways and neurotransmitters. This has prompted interest in antidepressant therapy as a treatment for chronic pain.

Systematic reviews of this approach were carried out at Water Reed Army Medical Center (2002) and University of Washington (2003). Researchers from both teams concluded that certain antidepressants provide modest pain relief in people with chronic back pain. The Washington team found that tricyclic and tetracyclic antidepressants were somewhat effective in relieving back pain, but that SSRIs (the class of antidepressants that includes Prozac, Paxil, and Zoloft) had no effect.

To date, only a few trials involving a small number of participants have examined the effect of antidepressant therapy on back pain. Additional and larger trials are needed before firm conclusions can be drawn.

Herbal Medicines

Several plant-based preparations have shown promise in the treatment of mild or occasional low back pain. A 2006 Cochrane Review found that derivatives of devil's claw, white willow bark, and cayenne all seemed to provide more short-term pain relief than placebo. However, researchers noted that existing studies are few and of poor methodological quality.

Additional research is therefore needed before any firm recommendations for or against herbal supplement therapy can be made.

Spinal Manipulative Therapy (SMT)

Spinal manipulative therapy refers to a variety of hands-on techniques that use touch pressure to relieve mechanical stress within the spine. SMT may be administered by a variety of professionals, including chiropractors, physical therapists, and osteopathic physicians. Many patients choose SMT because it's noninvasive, performed in outpatient settings, and has relatively few side effects.

Current research suggests that SMT provides modest, short-term benefits in people with both acute and chronic back pain. A 2003 meta-analysis conducted by the Cochrane Back Review Group found that SMT provided a slight decrease in pain intensity, but concluded that SMT showed no significant advantage over other common treatments like general practitioner care, analgesics, or exercise therapy. These results were further supported by a 2011 update, which was conducted by a multidisciplinary team and incorporated data from several recent, large-scale trials.

One advantage of SMT is its safety record. The Cochrane team found no evidence of serious complications among the 2011 trial participants. The most common side effects reported were mild and included muscle soreness, stiffness, and transient increase in pain.

The 2011 team concluded that SMT might have practical advantages over therapies of similar efficacy because of its relatively low cost, time-limited nature, and low risk of adverse effects. Decisions to pursue SMT, they wrote, should therefore be made on an individual basis, taking into account cost, available options, and patient and provider preference.

On a personal note, I have known some excellent SMT practitioners who have achieved positive outcomes for their patients. I've also seen many who provide standard, one-size-fits-all interventions rather than assessing and treating the root causes of patients' back problems. When choosing a chiropractor, it's very important to find someone who is both problem-focused and realistic about the limits of this type of therapy. A knowledgeable back specialist can often recommend a chiropractor who meets these criteria.

Physical Therapy

Physical therapy is a set of interventions designed to restore lost functioning in patients with disabling medical conditions. Components may include therapeutic exercise and movement, electrotherapy, ultrasound, heat and cold therapy, traction, and fitting of braces and supports. Many primary care providers prescribe physical therapy as a frontline treatment for low back pain.

Therapeutic Exercise

We previously discussed the probable benefits of staying active and maintaining a regular routine for patients with acute low back pain. By the same reasoning, might exercise help you recover even faster?

Research suggests not—at least not in the early stages. A 1995 study by Malmivaara and colleagues found that patients with acute lower back pain who were assigned back-mobilizing exercises had significantly more pain and less range of motion at three and twelve weeks follow-up than those who simply followed their normal routines. These findings were supported by a 2000 systematic review of thirty-nine separate trials. The team found strong evidence that exercise therapy during the acute stage was not any more effective than other treatments, including advice to simply stay active.

Conversely, research shows that a properly designed exercise therapy program can be an effective treatment for chronic lower back pain. In a 2005 systematic review at the University of Toronto, researchers identified several therapeutic practices that tended to improve patient outcomes. The most effective programs were generally tailored to the individual's medical needs, supervised by qualified therapists, and included both stretching and strengthening exercises.

The Toronto study results echo my own experience with physical therapy. I've encountered many excellent therapists who had the knowledge and clinical acumen to assess and treat specific biomechanical issues in their patients. However, too many therapists simply deliver standard back exercises that may or may not impact the root causes of the pain. There are also therapists who cling to the outdated notion that you shouldn't do exercise that hurts you. Taken too far, this approach can keep you from your daily activities, which actually hinders healing and normal functioning. A back specialist should be able to recommend an effective therapist who can meet your needs.

Transcutaneous Electrical Nerve Stimulation (TENS)

This common form of electrotherapy has been used for more than thirty years to treat chronic pain. TENS involves passing small, carefully modulated pulses of electricity through the skin. While the exact mechanism of action is disputed, this appears to inhibit the transmission of pain signals via the spinal cord. TENS is often prescribed as an adjunct to medication therapy and may be delivered by a physician, physical therapist, or at home by the patient.

The short- and long-term benefits of TENS are not well studied. While authoring a 2005 Cochrane Review, researchers identified thirty-nine published clinical trials of TENS, but excluded all but two due to methodological flaws. The remaining studies provided conflicting evidence regarding TENS' short-term effectiveness, and neither provided follow-up data. The team stressed the need for larger, more rigorous studies that followed patients' progress over time.

Traction

Traction for low back pain involves application of forces to stretch and elongate the back. In theory, this promotes healing by opening the z-joints and relieving pressure on the spinal cord and associated nerves and blood vessels. Force is usually applied gradually, by hand or with a system of weights and pulleys. Both physical therapists and chiropractors use this technique.

Existing research does not support traction as a stand-alone treatment for low back pain. A 2006 Cochrane Review found no evidence that traction alone was any more effective than sham treatment or no treatment. This held true for short- and long-term courses of therapy, various delivery types (continuous pressure versus intermittent), and patient characteristics (acute versus chronic pain). Researchers noted that due to methodological problems in existing studies, it was impossible to determine whether traction might be effective when used in conjunction with other interventions.

Complementary and Alternative Medicine (CAM)

CAM refers to a diverse group of practices, interventions, and products that fall outside the realm of conventional medicine as practiced by physicians, therapists, and allied health professionals. Common examples include herbal medicines, mind-body practices (meditation, progressive relaxation), acupuncture, massage, and traditional Chinese medicine. The 2007 National Health Interview Survey conducted by the National Institutes of Health found that about 38 percent of Americans use some form of CAM.

The line between conventional and alternative medicine is far from absolute. Many CAM therapies incorporate principals of conventional medicine, and some physicians and therapists recommend CAM as an adjunct to conventional treatments. While further research is needed to explore their benefits, risks, and cost-effectiveness, the following alternative therapies have shown promise in the treatment of chronic low back pain.

Acupuncture

Acupuncture is a form of traditional medicine that originated in ancient China and is used worldwide to treat pain and nausea. Acupuncturists insert solid needles through the skin in order to adjust the flow of psychic energy, or qi, throughout the body. Acupuncture points do not correspond to actual anatomical structures but rather to classical Eastern concepts of human function and vitality. A similar technique, dry-needling, involves the placement of needles at the source of the pain, which is called the trigger point.

A 2005 Cochrane Review found some evidence that acupuncture and dry-needling provide short-term pain relief and functional improvement in patients with chronic low back pain. Benefits were generally measurable immediately following the session and at one-week follow-up, but disappeared within a couple of weeks. Simultaneous treatment with acupuncture or dry-needling also appeared to enhance the benefits of conventional therapies such as exercise and non-narcotic painkillers, though such effects were small. A meta-analysis conducted the same year at the University of Maryland School of Medicine reached almost identical conclusions. However, larger, more rigorous studies are needed to support these findings.

Massage

Massage therapists use their hands (and sometimes mechanical devices) to manipulate muscle and connective tissue through the skin. Goals of massage therapy include pain relief, promotion of healing, and a sense of relaxation and well-being.

Results of a 2002 Cochrane Review suggested that massage therapy may be beneficial for people with subacute (medium duration) and chronic low back pain, especially when delivered in conjunction with therapeutic exercise and education. They also found some evidence that acupuncture massage, which combines tissue manipulation with needle placement, is more effective at relieving pain than massage alone. The team concluded that more research is needed to explore the longer-term benefits of massage as well as its cost-effectiveness.

Psychological Care

As I mentioned in chapter one, I rarely (if ever) see a patient whose back pain is caused by depression alone. However, I meet many people who have been referred for psychiatric evaluation because their pain appears to have no physical cause. Often this occurs when the doctor notices that the patient is depressed and concludes that the pain must therefore be psychogenic (originating in the mind).

It's true that back pain affects every part of your life—your career, relationships, and emotions. And because depression and physical pain share common biological pathways, one tends to intensify the other in a vicious cycle. I've seen people lose their jobs, become depressed, and hurt all over. I also remember one patient whose back pain vanished after her messy divorce concluded.

This isn't to suggest that pain is "all in your head." In a 2006 study published in Spine, researchers followed 5,211 recently injured whiplash patients for twelve months. None of the participants had a history of mental health problems. However, when they were examined six weeks after their injury, 42 percent reported symptoms of depression, and 37 percent of these experienced persistent or recurrent depression over the next year. These findings supported an earlier whiplash study by Radanov and colleagues in which 80 percent of the participants developed depression after their injuries, and 70 percent of these were still depressed two years later. Both teams concluded that the subjects' psychological problems were a consequence of their whiplash, not its cause.

That being said, research also shows that mental health care can play a positive role in the treatment of back pain. A 2007 meta-analysis conducted at Duke University Medical Center found robust evidence that patients treated with cognitive-behavioral or self-regulatory therapies experienced significant improvements in their pain intensity, quality of life, and mood. What's more, combining psychological care with other interventions like exercise and physical therapy helped patients return to work faster.

In my center, we sometimes refer patients to a psychologist or psychiatrist to help them cope with the emotional impact of their pain. However, we view counseling, behavioral intervention, and antidepressant therapy as parts of a comprehensive treatment plan—not solutions in themselves.

The Dangers of Untreated Back Pain: Mr. Jones' Downward Spiral

I've dedicated so much space to the topic of conservative care because I've seen too many patients who, like Mr. Jones, spiraled downward during months of ineffective treatments. Because they didn't understand their treatment options, they got caught in a self-perpetuating cycle of pain, depression, and physical deterioration.

Pain is a stressor that provokes your adrenal glands to release the stress-fighting hormone cortisol. When you have too much cortisol in your bloodstream for too long, your adrenal glands become depleted. This "adrenal fatigue" can cause you to feel extremely tired and run down. You may also experience muscle weakness, insomnia, depression, and headaches and crave salty, carbohydrate-rich foods.

All of these symptoms impact your health for the worse. Now, not only do you hurt, you feel sluggish, overweight, and out of shape. The resulting depression not only exacerbates your back pain, it eats away at your self-image, relationships, and ability to work. You feel like a failure. You see no hope in sight. So you get more depressed, which causes more pain and impairment.

For too many people, this downward spiral leads to chronic and sometimes indefinite narcotic use—reliance on opioids like Percocet, Oxycontin, and Dilaudid to relieve the pain. But while narcotics provide temporary relief, they can also deepen your depression by depleting your body's supply of mood-elevating chemicals (endorphins). So you start taking antidepressants too, which help your mood, but cause even more weight gain.

So what's at the bottom of Mr. Jones' downward spiral? To find out, let's fast-forward five years.

Mr. Jones comes into our center because he is unable to sleep through the night and can't walk or sit due to severe back pain that radiates down his legs. At this point, he's tried everything: narcotics, St. John's wort, epidural steroid injections, physical therapy, even back surgery. Nothing has worked for long.

Fortunately, he proves to be a good candidate for treatment with a spinal cord stimulator (more on this later). Testing after trial implantation shows that his pain has vanished. We're heartened by his positive response and consider his case a success.

Yet when Mr. Jones and his wife return for a follow-up appointment, he's unhappy. Though he admits he's sleeping well and able to do what he wants, he's now complaining about a new kind of back pain. The insertion site where the stimulator was implanted is still bothering him, he says. What can we do to help?

Sadly, nothing. I don't believe patients like Mr. Jones consciously want to be unhappy or in pain, but they've become so habituated to narcotics, so shrouded in emotional troubles, and so accustomed to disability, they no longer knew how to function as well people. Perhaps Mr. Jones also gets some secondary benefits—attentive caregiving from his wife, an exemption from the stresses of work—that will disappear if he recovers. I wouldn't go so far as to say that he's past the point of no return, but his prognosis is poor indeed.

Key Points

- If you or someone you care about has been living with back pain for two months or longer, consider Mr. Jones' story a cautionary tale. Don't wait for it to become chronic. Rather than jumping through more hoops (physical therapy, pain management with opioids), consider consulting a spine specialist who can explain your full range of options.
- If you already feel yourself spiraling downward, know that this pattern is reversible. With solution-focused treatment, you can improve your depression, activity level, and muscle strength—and this can help reduce your pain.

In the next few chapters, we'll delve deeper into some common causes of back pain and procedures that offer hope for lasting relief.

4

DISC PAIN: AN INVISIBLE MENACE

Christy, age forty, already had a long history of back pain before things took a turn for the worse in 2009. Ever since her twenties, her back had been acting up every few months. The pain was usually dull and achy and centered over the lower part of her spine. "I figured I was just sitting too much," says Christy, who worked a desk job at an insurance company before her sons were born.

Usually, a few Tylenol did the trick during her flare-ups. However, twice the pain had gotten so bad she'd seen a specialist, who treated her with epidural steroid injections. In both cases the discomfort eased, but Christy was never sure if it was the steroids that helped or something else.

Shortly after her twin sons were born, Christy went through her worst episode of back pain yet—and this time it stuck around. Mothering twins, she soon learned, involved a lot of heavy lifting. As the kids grew, she developed buff biceps that her friends envied. But at the same time, her back pain intensified.

Christy's doctor said her x-rays and MRI looked fine and prescribed physical therapy. He made a comment that being an "older mother" must be tough on her body. "I was furious," Christy says. "I knew there was something more to it. I felt as though he wasn't taking my concerns seriously."

When her boys were two, Christy formed a toddler playgroup with a couple of other moms in the neighborhood. Meetings were supposed to rotate between the members' homes, but Christy never volunteered. By now, her pain was so severe that it was all she could do to dress, feed, and bathe her kids. Housework beyond occasional dusting was out of the question. When the group decided to walk to the park a few blocks away, she begged off knowing she'd never make it that far pushing a stroller.

After a solid year of physical therapy failed to do the trick, Christy's doctor referred her to pain management. "I thought I'd finally get some answers," she says. "Instead, they started talking about putting me on oxycodone and hydrocodone. I thought, 'Seriously, how am I supposed to chase two boys around the house when I'm zoned out on narcotics?'" She fired her doctors and came to our center for a second opinion.

Christy brought her imaging studies to our first appointment, and indeed, her discs looked fairly healthy. She wondered aloud if maybe the problem were all in her head. I assured her that even powerful technology like MRI often misses what's happening inside a disc. To look for hidden problems, I performed a procedure called disc stimulation in which contrast dye is slowly and carefully injected into the discs to raise their internal pressure and stretch the outer annulus. When painful tears are present, the procedure provokes discomfort. The pain is deemed concordant when the patient's usual pain location is reproduced and discordant if the pain is not in that location. Sure enough, Christy experienced sharp pain in the typical location of her pain when one of her discs were pressurized, which suggested a common and essentially invisible condition called internal disc disruption syndrome. It's invisible because one can't inspect the appearance of a disc and make that diagnosis purely based on its observation.

Disc Pain: What Is It?

Disc problems are a common cause of low back pain accounting for about 40 percent of all cases. But while the condition itself is well studied, it can be quite difficult to treat. Too often, physicians prolong conservative therapy because they don't realize that other options are available.

In this chapter, we'll examine the origins of disc pain and create a roadmap for accurate diagnosis. We'll also discuss treatment options—both those currently available and a few that appear promising for the near future.

Common Disc Conditions

As you'll recall from Chapter 2, the intervertebral discs lie between the vertebral bodies and provide cushioning and limited movement to the spine. They consist of a gel-like inner core called the nucleus pulposus surrounded by multiple rings of ligament that form the annulus fibrosus. Two cartilage endplates join the disc faces to the adjacent vertebrae.

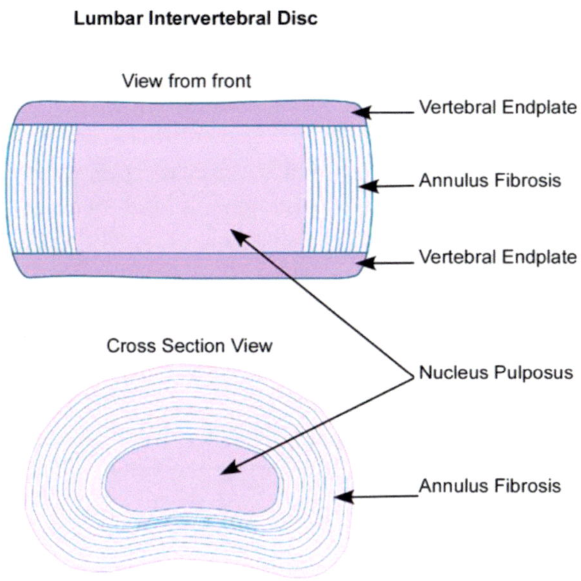

Figure 7

Disc Degeneration

As we age, our discs naturally begin to show signs of wear and tear. The term "degeneration" generally refers to changes like annular tears, reduced disc height, a misshaped nucleus, or loss and dehydration of the nuclear material. Many of these changes are evident on routine imaging studies and may even be discovered by accident.

Hearing that you have degenerated discs can be frightening, but don't let it worry you too much. An extensive body of research shows no definitive correlation between disc degeneration and back pain. In fact, the condition appears to be very common in people who are pain-free. For this reason, pioneering spine pain specialist Nikolai Bogduk, MD, of the University of New Castle in Australia, has suggested that physicians use the less distressing term "normal age changes" when discussing disc degeneration with patients.

While degeneration is often painless, discomfort may result if a tear within the annulus allows nuclear material to spread outward. The nucleus pulposus is rich in nerve-irritating substances called algogens and inflammatory mediators. If these reach the nociceptors (pain-sensing nerve endings) in the outer annulus, pain can result. This in turn increases the sensitivity of the nociceptors, which causes even more discomfort.

In addition to heightening pain sensitivity, annular tears may also provide a pathway for the ingrowth of blood vessels and nerves. In a healthy disc, only the outer third of the annulus is innervated. However, nerve endings sometimes grow into areas where it doesn't belong. This process, called "neoinnervation," appears to play an important role in the generation of low back pain.

In one recent study, British researchers at the University of Manchester examined tissue samples from discs removed during back surgery. All samples were confirmed to be herniated (bulging) to the point where they put pressure on the spinal nerves. In 46 percent of these samples, nerve endings had invaded the inner layers of the annulus, and in 21 percent, they extended into the nucleus. When stimulated in the laboratory, the invasive nerve endings expressed the pain-producing neurotransmitter Substance P. Researchers concluded that neoinnervation might therefore be an important contributing factor in some cases of chronic low back pain.

Internal Disc Disruption (IDD) Syndrome

This condition occurs when the disc annulus develops tears called radial fissures that project out from the center of the disc like spokes on a wheel. Because these internal tears are not always detectable by MRI, the disc may appear normal on imaging studies. Furthermore, these tears aren't always painful. Even when present, they may or may not be causing the actual back pain that you have been living with.

Trouble usually begins when the vertebral endplate, which seals the disc against the adjacent bone, fractures due to trauma or repetitive stress. This causes the nucleus to lose the internal pressure that allows it to bear weight and distribute force evenly. Pressure within the disc becomes uneven and shifts to the rear—which happens to be the area of the disc richest in nocioceptors.

Endplate failure also kicks off an inflammatory response, which upsets certain processes in the nucleus pulposus. Inflammation inhibits the production of proteins called proteoglycans, which bind water to the nuclear material and regulate transport between cells. Without them, the nucleus begins to dehydrate. Cells starve and die off from lack of nutrients, leading to the build-up of waste products like lactic acid. Over time, the soft, gel-like matrix is replaced with tough, fibrous cartilage.

As the nucleus degrades, the annulus begins to crack from the inside out. The resulting inflammation heightens pain sensitivity along the tears and promotes the growth of fibrous scar tissue. The severity of IDD syndrome is graded by the extent of these annular fissures. In their early stages, they may impact only the inner layer of the annulus. As they grow, they eventually reach the outer layers and may begin to extend outward beneath the disc surface.

When tearing reaches the nerve endings in the outer annulus, pain may result. (This can happen even earlier in highly innervated discs.) Patients experience lumbar IDD syndrome as persistent pain of the low back that typically (but not always) worsens with prolonged sitting or repetitive bending. Lying down or standing often eases the discomfort.

Disc Herniation

In some cases, the nucleus pulposus migrates along annular tears, creating bulges or bumps in the disc surface. When large enough, these can press on nearby nerve roots, causing leg pain and neurological symptoms. In severe cases, the nucleus may actually protrude through a tear in the disc surface, causing chemical as well as mechanical irritation to the nerves.

While related to IDD syndrome, disc herniation requires quite different treatments, which are discussed in detail in Chapter 7.

Causes of Disc Pain

Age appears to be the strongest risk factor for disc degeneration. Genetic factors, such as the ability to produce certain protective proteins and bone substances also play a role. In rare cases, a metabolic disease like diabetes can weaken the spinal structure and accelerate degeneration.

IDD syndrome again, appears to begin with disc endplate failure, which is most commonly due to repetitive stress. Studies show that this can happen after as few as one hundred repetitions at just 50 to 60 percent of the disc's ultimate tensile strength (in other words, the amount of force needed to tear it). Such forces can occur during everyday activity like moving furniture, shoveling snow, or yard work.

Diagnosis

To treat discogenic pain, your physician must first identify the specific disc or discs that are causing the problem. This can be difficult, because in many cases, the damage lies within the body of the disc and may not appear on imaging studies.

Diagnosis is complicated by the fact that some signs of disc degeneration like annular tears and loss of disc height do register on x-rays and MRIs. Physicians sometimes assume that the most degraded disc must be the source of discomfort. However, as noted above, research shows no clear correlation between disc degeneration and pain.

Lumbar Disc Stimulation

Lumbar disc stimulation, often called discography, is a minimally invasive procedure that is considered the gold standard in IDD syndrome diagnosis. Think of it as your doctor reaching inside your back, tapping on a disc, and asking, "Is this where it usually hurts?"

During disc stimulation, contrast fluid is injected directly into the nucleus of the discs. Pressure is carefully monitored with a gauge and increased until it either causes pain or reaches the cut-off threshold. For the test to be positive, the resulting pain should feel similar to your normal back pain. Afterward, your doctor may take a CT scan of your spine.

IDD syndrome is generally diagnosed when:

- Disc stimulation reproduces your usual back pain
- The pain evoked is at least a 7 on a 10-point pain intensity scale
- Pain is reproduced by repeated injections at the same pressure
- Stimulation of adjacent discs is painless
- A CT scan reveals extensive fissures within the annulus

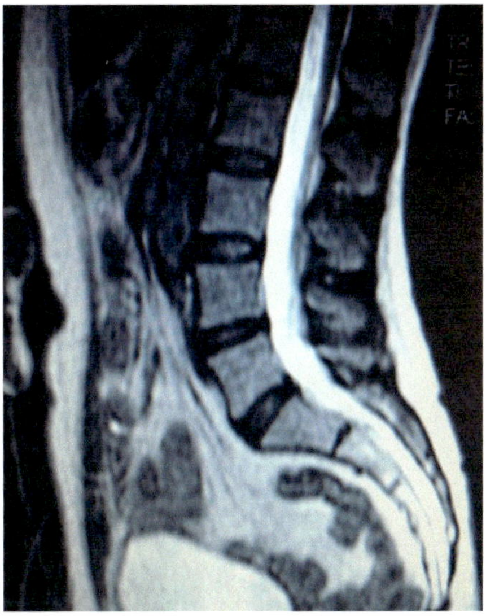

Figure 8: This spinal MRI of a forty-nine-year-old male with chronic back pain shows very mild degenerative changes of the lower two discs. The patient later underwent disc stimulation (shown below).

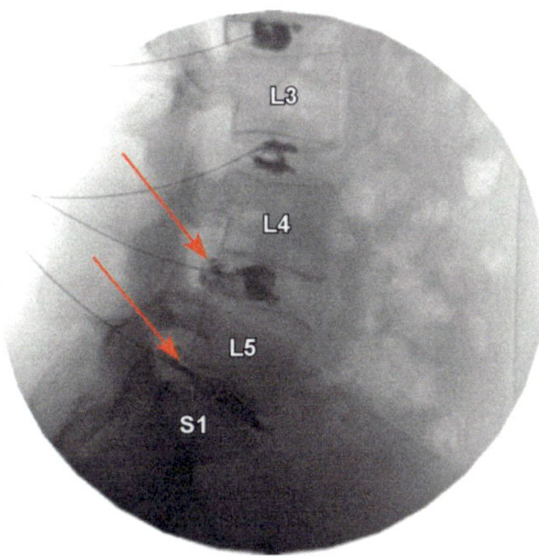

Figure 9: Imaging after disc stimulation demonstrated a annular tears that were not visible on MRI. Interestingly, the tears were not painful with pressure stimulation.

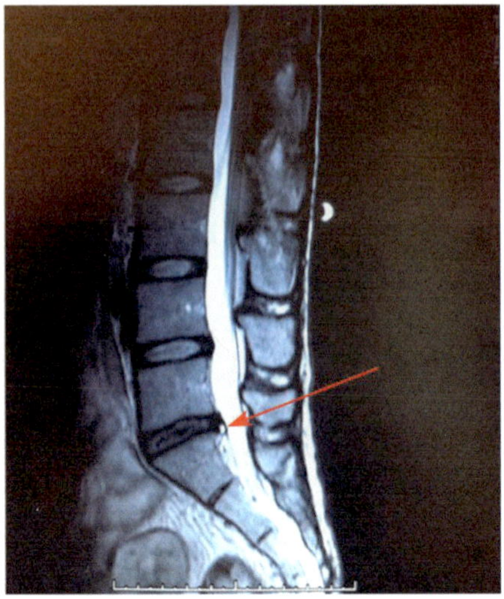

Figure 10: Note the high intensity zone at L5/1.

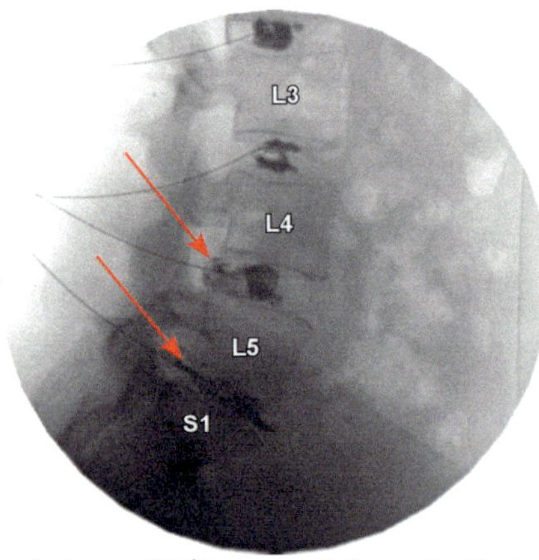

Figure 11: Disc stimulation at L5/1 recreated the patient's typical low back pain. The annular tears at L4/5 were painless.

Does disc stimulation work?

Disc stimulation has weathered some controversy, though many of the concerns raised have been disproved by research. The latest evidence suggests that it's an extremely reliable diagnostic test when performed by a properly trained professional and according to established clinical guidelines.

Results of a 1968 study by Earl P. Holt suggested a high false-positive rate for disc stimulation. In other words, the test routinely detected IDD syndrome when it didn't exist. However, Holt's experiment had serious methodological flaws. Most importantly, he didn't use a gauge to measure and control injection pressure. Even a healthy disc will hurt if the internal stress is raised high enough, which may explain why his team observed so many "false positives."

Holt's findings have since been roundly debunked. In one study, interventional pain management pioneer Richard Derby, MD, pressurized the discs of healthy patients to the diagnostic threshold for IDD syndrome as set forth in the published guidelines of the International Spine Intervention Society. None of these patients reported pain. A 2003 study of 4,319 patients by Kevin Pauza, MD, and colleagues found a very low false-positive rate (approximately 1 percent) for disc stimulation performed by a skilled physician following accepted protocols. These findings and others suggest that disc stimulation is indeed a useful tool for pinpointing a particular disc as a pain source.

Eugene Carragee and colleagues raised a more recent alarm after completing a ten-year longitudinal study on disc stimulation in 2000. Carragee's results suggested the procedure might actually accelerate disc degeneration, leading to high rates of herniation decreased disc heights, and other degenerative changes. Once again, the work had a number of serious methodological flaws. First, nearly 40 percent of the subjects dropped out during the study, and it stands to reason that the remainder represented those with the most severe back pain. This "self-selection" effect likely skewed results in favor of patients with severe disc disease, which may not have been caused by disc stimulation. Additionally, Carragee's conclusions are unique. There is no other evidence that the procedure, which has been around for decades, has any harmful long-term effects.

Is disc stimulation right for you?

This test is generally appropriate for patients with back pain that is chronic and unresponsive to standard conservative care. To benefit from the procedure, you must be able to communicate effectively with your physician and accurately describe any pain that occurs during pressurization. You should not undergo this test if you are pregnant or have signs of spine infection (such as a fever or a history of IV drug use).

In many cases, your physician will order a screening MRI before proceeding with disc stimulation. MRI can sometimes pick up direct signs of disc disruption, which are helpful to know before pressurization. "High intensity zones," which appear as bright spots on the back part of the disc wall, may indicate nuclear material that has migrated along a radial fissure. MRI also occasionally detects certain lesions characteristic of endplate rupture. However, the fact that an MRI is "negative" for disc problems should not rule out the need for disc stimulation.

What to expect

Disc stimulation can be performed in a well-equipped physician's office, outpatient surgery center, or hospital. Injections are typically administered by a doctor while a nurse or other assistant records your responses. Often a technologist will also be in the room operating the fluoroscope, which allows the physician to visualize the needle under x-ray guidance.

Before the procedure, your doctor will explain how to rate your pain on a 0-10 scale. You'll also be asked to indicate whether the pain produced by pressurization is similar to your usual back pain.

Before each injection, the skin and tissue above the target disc is numbed with local anesthetic. If pressurization provokes your typical pain, your doctor will repeat the procedure a short time later to confirm the findings. In some cases, local anesthetic is injected afterward to relieve any lingering discomfort.

After disc stimulation, the technologist might take a CT scan of your spine. The contrast agent within your discs will show the location and extent of any radial tears. Imaging also confirms that the contrast agent has been properly placed within the disc nuclei.

Aftercare

After disc stimulation, you'll need to spend thirty minutes under observation. Common side effects include back pain, which may increase over the next few days. Your doctor may prescribe painkillers to take as needed. While complications are rare, call your physician if your pain is severe or can't be relieved with medication.

Treatments for Disc Pain

Once a diagnosis of IDD syndrome is confirmed, several treatment options are available, including steroid injections. In addition, some patients still benefit from electrothermal annuloplasty, though this is not as popular as it used to be.. Promising biologic treatments are also being studied, and at least one is currently available. Surgery, another possible option, will be discussed in detail in Chapter 9.

Epidural Steroid Injections

For some patients, steroid injections near a painful disc can provide temporary relief and improve quality of life. Corticosteroids are medications with strong inflammation-fighting properties. In theory, they prevent the release of pain-transmitting chemicals and reduce swelling and discomfort in the torn annulus. Common examples include methylprednisolone and triamcinolone.

To relieve disc pain, steroids are typically injected into the anterior (front) portion of the epidural space (the hollow area between the disc and spinal nerves) directly beside the painful disc. Considerable skill is required in order to deliver the medication to precisely the right spot without harming nerves or other structures. It is therefore mandatory that these procedures be performed under fluoroscopic guidance by a trained and experienced physician.

Corticosteroids can be delivered by one of two routes. Interlaminar injections place the medication into the lumbar epidural space, while transforaminal injections target the junction of the disc and spinal nerve via the neural foramen. Of the two, the transforaminal route is better supported by research, but requires significantly more skill and training to administer safely. If you're unsure of your physician's educational background, don't hesitate to ask before agreeing to the procedure.

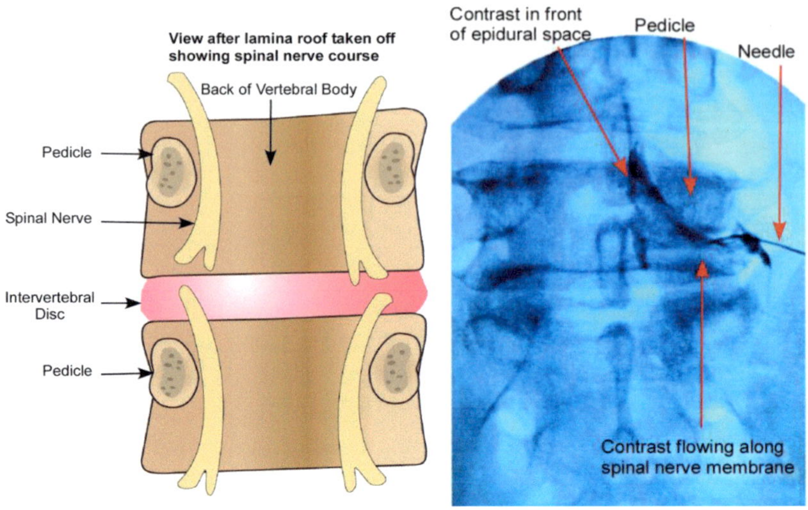

Figure 13: A spinal needle within the sheath of the exiting spinal nerve shown on the right in an actual patient in an L5 transforaminal epidural steroid injection. Note the contrast material flow along the spinal nerve into the regional epidural space underneath the pedicle.

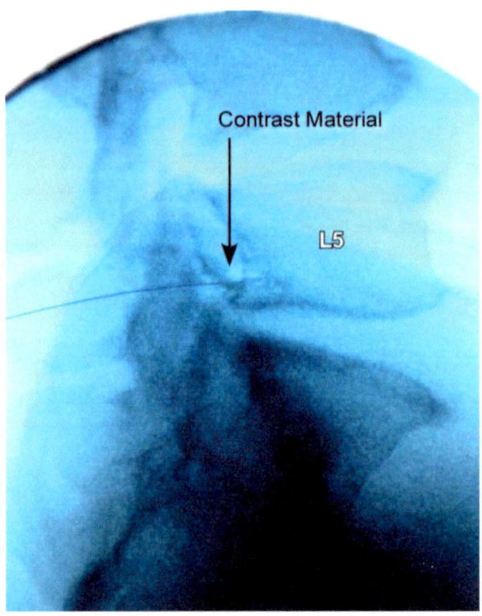

Figure 14: Note the dark contrast in front of the needle, which is positioned behind the L5 vertebral body.

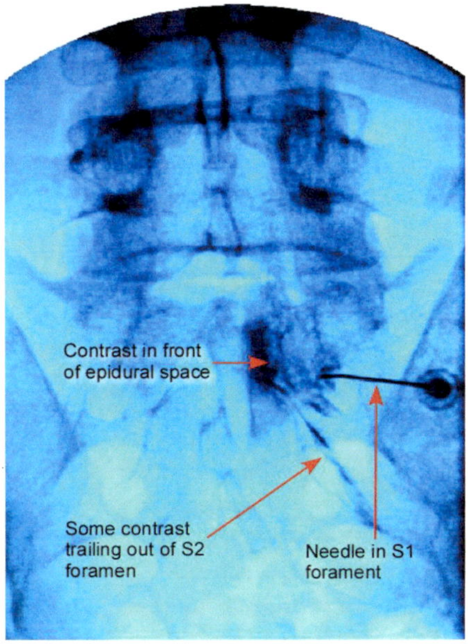

Figure 15: Transforaminal epidural steroid injection at S1 on the right for right low back pain confirmed to be from the L5/1 disc with disc stimulation.

Do epidural steroid injections work?

Preliminary evidence suggests that steroid injections can be a cost-effective alternative to surgery for some people with discogenic pain. A 2009 Korean study involving patients with disc herniation found that both interlaminar and transforaminal injections provided significant pain relief at both two weeks and four months follow up. However, additional trials are needed to bolster these findings.

Are epidural steroid injections right for me?

A trial corticosteroid injection may be appropriate if you have discogenic pain confirmed by disc stimulation.

Risks and side effects

The most common side effect is a brief headache, which occurs in about 3 percent of patients. Serious complications are rare and include injury to the arteries or spinal cord. Injections can also cause bleeding; tell your doctor if you have a clotting disorder or are taking blood thinning medications or NSAIDs.

What to expect

The procedure is performed on an x-ray-sensitive table. You will typically lie face down over a curved surface that opens the joints of your back. A nurse or technician may administer light IV sedation to help you relax. Before the injection, the skin and tissue over the disc will be numbed with a local anesthetic. The needle is then inserted under x-ray guidance until it reaches the target area in the epidural space. Your doctor will first inject a small amount of dye to verify correct needle placement and finish with a mixture of steroid and numbing medication.

Aftercare

If you were sedated during the procedure, you'll probably feel drowsy. Avoid driving or operating machinery for at least twelve hours. You may also notice some numbness or tingling in your legs. This usually disappears in a day or two. In most cases, you will be able to resume your normal activities the next day.

Methylene Blue Injections: One to Watch

Several years ago, researchers began to explore a possible alternative to steroid injections. Methylene blue (MB) is a chemical compound commonly prescribed to treat urinary tract infections as well as certain blood disorders. It's also used as an injectable contrast agent that improves the sharpness and quality of x-rays and other imaging studies.

A single MB injection directly into a painful intervertebral disc has been proposed to have therapeutic benefits in some people with chronic discogenic back pain. While its exact mechanism of action is unknown, MB is believed to help to reduce levels of nitric oxide, which in turn inhibits immune response and reduces inflammation. Because MB is mildly toxic to the nerves, it might also kill nerve endings that have invaded the disc and are sensing painful injuries deep inside.

A small clinical trial of intradiscal MB injection was conducted in China in 2007 that demonstrated results that have not been reproducible. All twenty-four participants had chronic discogenic pain confirmed by disc stimulation and met the criteria for spinal fusion surgery. At one to two years follow up, 90 percent of the subjects were either completely pain free or felt so much better that they no longer needed painkillers. These dramatic results caused much excitement among back pain experts, who were keen to see if these successes could be replicated on a larger scale.

Unfortunately, subsequent trials of the treatment have been less positive. In 2012, Korean researchers trialed single intradiscal MB injection in a group of twenty participants with confirmed discogenic pain. At three months follow up, 55 percent showed marked improvement. However, at one year follow-up, only 20 percent were still experiencing significant relief.

Intradiscal Electrothermal Annuloplasty (IDET)

IDET uses electrically generated heat energy to destroy nociceptors in the outer disc annulus and interrupt the transmission of pain signals to the brain. Under fluoroscopic guidance, the physician inserts a hollow needle into the rear side of the annulus and threads a catheter with a heating element through it. The catheter is slowly heated to 90 degrees Celsius (194 degrees Fahrenheit) and left at maximum temperature for about four minutes. The heat application is carefully controlled and does not harm the spinal nerves or surrounding tissue.

Does IDET work?

To date, no systematic review of IDET's efficacy has been produced. However, studies suggest benefits in carefully selected patient groups. In a randomized, controlled trial involving sixty-four patients with confirmed discogenic low back pain, IDET produced statistically significant reduction in pain intensity. Before the study, all subjects were carefully screened for depression, significant loss of disc height, recent surgical intervention, and other potentially confounding conditions. While this study is believed to be the most representative to date, further research is needed to clarify the treatment's benefits and limitations.

Is IDET right for you?

IDET may be appropriate if:

- You have disc pain confirmed by disc stimulation
- Your pain lasts at least three months
- You haven't had prior back surgeries at the affected level
- MRI shows no signs of disc herniation

Risks and side effects

IDET is generally safe, and long-term complications are rare. Possible risks include heat injury to the surrounding tissues and nerve punctures. Mild punctures usually need no intervention, though they may cause a brief headache. More severe punctures may require surgical repair and could result in lasting disability.

What to expect

The procedure is usually performed on an x-ray-sensitive table under fluoroscopic guidance. After administering a mild sedative, the physician numbs the puncture site with local anesthetic. The needle and probe are inserted through the skin into the disc annulus and heated slowly to the recommended temperature. After cauterization, additional antibiotics and painkillers may be injected into the disc to prevent infection and minimize discomfort.

Aftercare

Following IDET, you may notice a slight increase in your back pain for a few days. This can usually be treated with over-the-counter pain medications.

The full benefits of IDET may take several weeks to appear. During this time, you will be advised to stay active and may be given exercises to perform at home. However, you should avoid heavy lifting or prolonged sitting for eight to twelve weeks and athletics for several months. Your doctor will let you know when it's safe to increase your activity level. Once you're fully healed, physical therapy may be prescribed to help restore your strength and range of motion.

Biologic Treatments

Biologics are therapeutic substances created by biological rather than chemical processes. Familiar examples include vaccines, blood products, antibodies, and transplantable tissues grown from stem cells. Biologic approaches are especially exciting because they have the potential to permanently reverse the effects of IDD syndrome and restore degenerated discs to health. Potential benefits include:

- Reversal of matrix degeneration within the nucleus

- Inhibition of harmful inflammatory chemicals
- Repair of existing tissue fissures and injury
- Restoration of optimal hydration, oxygenation, and pH balance

As of early 2013, all of the following treatments are still under investigation. An exception is the Biostat System fibrin sealant, which is publically available.

Direct injections.

In a healthy disc, certain proteins play a crucial role in the production of nuclear and annular material. During IDD syndrome, inflammation and cell death deplete these crucial proteins to dangerously low levels. Injecting lab-cultivated versions of these substances directly into the diseased disc has been shown to reinvigorate production, which can stop and even reverse the early effects of disc disease. Benefits such as increased disc height, reduced inflammation, and increased proteoglycan density have been observed in some animal trials.

The following proteins show the most promise as therapeutic agents. Administering several together as a "cocktail" may further increase their benefits:

- Osteogenic proteins
- Bone morphogenic proteins (BMPs)
- Sox-9
- Tissue inhibitor of metalloproteinase-1 (TIMP-1)
- Platelet-rich plasma (derived from the patient's own blood)

Direct gene therapy

When therapeutic proteins are injected directly, they are eventually used up or eliminated from the disc tissue. A more sustainable solution is to stimulate the disc to produce its own supply of these substances. This can be accomplished by inserting certain protein-synthesizing genes into existing disc cells.

One way to transfer therapeutic genes is by incorporating them into a virus (which has been genetically altered so that it can't cause disease). When the virus is injected into the disc, it "infects" the target cells and inserts its own DNA into them. Hence the infected cells now produce therapeutic proteins, and so do their "offspring" after division.

Viral delivery models for gene therapy are currently under investigation in animal trials and limited human trials. Several have resulted in the expression of protein-synthesizing genes, and one has even been shown to restore lost disc height in animals. However, more research is needed to understand and prevent potentially fatal immune responses before human trials expand.

Cell therapy

This process involves the transplantation of healthy cells into a diseased disc for the purpose of regenerating lost tissue. In the future, it could be used to treat cases of advanced IDD syndrome where extensive cell death has occurred. The most abundant source of new "seed" cells comes from stem cells, which are harvested from the patient's own bone marrow.

Stem cells are pluripotent, meaning they can transform into many other cell types as they grow. They can be cultivated into disc cells through exposure to BMPs or healthy disc cells harvested from the patient. Additional genetic manipulations may be necessary to help the transplant cells survive in the oxygen- and nutrient-poor environment of the diseased disc. Once the new cells are plentiful enough, they are injected into the disc, where they divide and repopulate the damaged matrix.

Limited cell therapy studies have been carried out in humans, and the FDA is currently studying the safety and efficacy of the procedure.

Tissue engineering

Scientists can now create tissues to replace those lost to IDD syndrome. One example that is currently available to patients is the Biostat System, a fibrin sealant heavily researched by Kevin Pauza, MD. Fibrin sealant is made of the blood plasma derivatives fibrinogen and thrombin, which work together to promote clotting. Similar sealants are used to treat organ and spinal cord trauma and stop uncontrolled bleeding.

When injected into the disc, Biostat seals up annular fissures. This blocks the release of pain chemicals from the affected nerve endings, reducing inflammatory response and halting degradation of the surrounding nuclear matrix. In the absence of irritating chemicals and reactions, the disc is more likely to heal itself and respond favorably to additional biologic treatments.

In 2013, Pauza presented results of a five-year Biostat trial at the North American Spine Society New Technology Summit. Participants included twenty-five patients who had undergone failed spinal fusion surgery for chronic disc pain. Most had exhausted the available treatment options and were at serious risk of long-term pain and disability. At the beginning of the study, their reported back pain intensity averaged 8.1 on a 0-10 scale. Five years after treatment with Biostat, this number had dropped to 4.0.

As of this writing, Biostat is available from Pauza's private practice at the Texas Spine and Joint Hospital in Tyler, Texas. The transplant takes about five minutes and is performed under local anesthetic. Some patients notice a temporary increase in back pain and discomfort afterward that can last for several weeks, but usually goes away on its own as the body adjusts to the new disc height.

Christy: One Hundred Percent Mom Again

After her IDD diagnosis, Christy and her husband discussed the pros and cons of surgery and decided it offered the best hope for lasting relief. Last year she underwent spinal fusion (which we'll discuss further in Chapter 9) and has been very pleased with the results. "I was nervous about being out of commission for so long, but I was also getting to the point where I felt like I was failing my kids," she says. "I had been dealing with this their entire lives. They needed their mom to be there one hundred percent."

Today, Christy feels better than ever and juggles parenting, housework, playgroup, and volunteering at her kids' cooperative preschool. Like many people who undergo back surgery, she has some residual pain but can control it with over-the-counter medications.

In retrospect, she's happy she followed her gut and sought out better care. "Firing my first doctor was scary, but it was the right choice," she says. "I was really surprised to find out how little the average physician knows about back pain.

"If you feel your doctor's not listening or taking the wrong approach, don't be afraid to speak up. Doctors have a lot of expertise, but they're not gods. Sometimes they don't recognize their own limitations."

Key Points:

- Wear and tear of the discs is normal as we age and isn't necessarily painful or a reason for concern. However, in a small number of cases, these degenerative changes can cause considerable discomfort.
- Failure of the disc's endplate can result in painful internal disc disruption (IDD) syndrome, leading to significant pain and functional loss.
- Imaging studies often miss signs of IDD syndrome. Disc stimulation is required for a definitive diagnosis.
- Once the painful disc is identified, the condition can be treated by a variety of means, including corticosteroid injections, IDET, and surgery.
- Experimental biologic therapies have shown great promise for the treatment of IDD syndrome. One of these, the Biostat System, is currently available to the public.

The discs aren't the only possible source of simple low back pain. In the next chapter we'll look at another common cause: the zygopophyseal or z-joints.

5

ZYGAPOPHYSEAL JOINT PAIN: THE FACTS ON SPINAL ARTHRITIS

He was in his forties, too young to retire. But his job as a long-haul truck driver was taking a toll on his back. "For fourteen years, I sat behind the wheel for most of the week," Marvin says. When he reached his destination, he'd help with the unloading, which required a good deal of bending, lifting, and twisting.

The pain came on gradually, starting at the bottom of his spine and eventually radiating to his buttocks. Sitting seemed to make it worse. After a few hours of driving, he was so sore he could barely climb out of his cab.

At his family doctor's recommendation, Marvin saw a chiropractor every weekend and went through several courses of physical therapy. He even took up yoga and practiced religiously on the road (though he knew he looked pretty funny doing tree poses beside his rig). Still, the pain worsened to the point that he had to limit himself to local assignments, which cut his income in half.

Finally his physician referred him to a pain management doctor, who gave him cortisone shots on either side of his back. That helped for a month or so, but then the pain came right back. They tried an epidural steroid injection, which didn't help either. When the doctor tried to prescribe him the narcotic Vicodin, Marvin resisted. "I was having a tough enough time hanging on to my job," he says. "When you're driving, you need to be alert. Also, my employer can and does drug test me at any time. I knew I'd never pass with that stuff in my system."

When a family friend recommended our center, Marvin didn't want to go at first. He was afraid that he'd just be disappointed again. But he couldn't keep going on the way he was—in pain and increasingly broke.

At his first appointment, he broke down in tears. "If you can't help him, please tell us now," said his wife. "And help us get to someone who can."

Marvin brought along some x-ray films that had been ordered by his family doctor. These showed enlargement of several of his back joints, including visible bone spurs on one. While such changes are common as we age, I decided to investigate further. In the meantime, I prescribed a non-narcotic painkiller called tramadol to keep him comfortable until we could find and treat the root cause of the problem.

At our next appointment, I had Marvin lie facedown on the x-ray table and used a fluoroscope to inject a short-acting anesthetic around the medial branch nerves that carried sensory signals between the suspicious-looking joint and his spinal cord. Once he was numb, I had him go through all the motions that normally hurt his back—sitting and bending forward as if to lift a crate. His back pain was gone.

Though Marvin's pain soon returned when the anesthetic wore off, I told him his response was promising. "We need to repeat the test in order to be sure," I told him, "but I think we just found an important clue as to what might be causing the problem." And that, of course, was the first step toward recovery.

What Is Z-Joint Pain?

Zygopophyseal joint (or z-joint) pain is common, accounting for 15 to 40 percent of all chronic low back pain cases. Patients—and even physicians—often mistake it for disc pain because there are no clear-cut imaging or physical examination findings that can diagnose it. Though joint and disc pain often feel similar, they respond in predictable ways to completely different diagnostic tests and treatments.

As you'll recall from Chapter 3, your z-joints lie between your lumbar vertebrae, just behind the main body of your spinal column. Each intervertebral level contains two joints located on either side of your backbone. Together with the discs, these structures give your lower back its flexibility, allowing you to bend, stretch and twist.

Whenever your z-joints move, the facets (bones) that comprise each joint slide smoothly over one another. In healthy joints, these surfaces are coated with moist cartilage, and the joint itself is contained within a capsule filled with synovial fluid. Both the cartilage and fluid provide lubrication that helps the joint function smoothly.

The outer part of the joint capsule is rich in nerve endings, which are linked directly to your spinal column via the small sensory fibers called medial branch nerves. These nerves transmit sensory information, including pain and pressure, from the facet joint to your central nervous system. They are also partially responsible for the contraction of little muscles called multifidi that help support your spine.

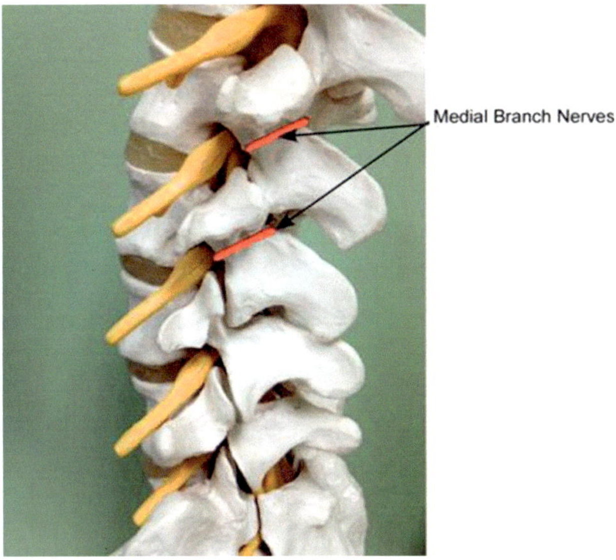

Figure 16

As we age, some of our discs naturally shrink and degenerate, which increases pressure on the bony surfaces of the z-joints. When this happens, the bones step up their production of bony matrix, resulting in enlargement (hypertrophy) of the joint and the formation of callous-like spurs along the facet edges. (This change is similar to what happens to your hands when you work all summer in the yard. Your skin responds to the extra stress by producing callouses—patches of tough, protective skin.) In your back, excess force and structural irregularities can gradually wear away the protective joint cartilage, causing z-joint arthropathy (also known as osteoarthritis).

Arthritis of the back appears to be very common. Often, it's painless and diagnosed by accident when the person undergoes imaging studies for an unrelated condition. Results of one cadaver study suggests that the spines of nearly 60 percent of people ages twenty to twenty-nine already show some arthritic changes.

In some cases, arthritis causes the z-joints to become painful. This can provoke spasms in nearby muscles, which leads to secondary pain and stiffness. Symptoms of z- joint pain differ widely from person to person. Although some textbooks describe the pain as being worsened by bending backwards (which compresses the joint and increases the pressure within), that's not always the case. In some people, bending forward is actually more painful because it stretches the joint capsule. Additionally, pain when twisting and bending sideways can indicate z-joint problems.

Arthritis-related back pain usually comes on gradually, though it may appear suddenly in cases of trauma. Often, it lingers for a while, then subsides for months or even years. The condition may follow an episodic course with occasional flare-ups and periods of normalcy between.

Z-joint pain doesn't usually radiate below the knee, though some people notice pain or tingling in the buttocks or the backs of the thighs. An exception is when a bone spur compresses the spinal cord or nerve root. This condition, also known as spinal stenosis, can cause severe leg pain as well as weakness, numbness, and slowed reflexes in the legs. For more information, see Chapter 8.

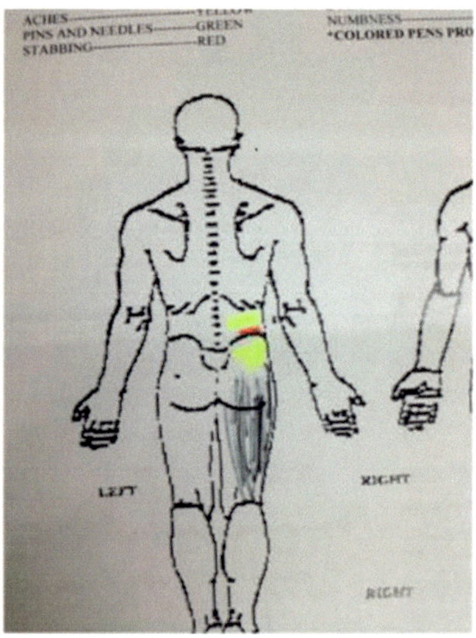

Figure 17: Pain drawing by a patient whose symptoms originated in the L4/5 and L5/1 z-joints. Her pain resolved completely after radiofrequency neurotomy of the respective medial branch nerves.

Diagnosis

Before recommending a structure-specific treatment, your physician needs to confirm that your pain is due to z-joint issues—and also to identify which joint or joints are causing the problem. Again, no specific history or physical examination findings can reliably differentiate z-joint pain from other types of discomfort like disc pain. While imaging studies may reveal bone spurs and other structural changes, these findings don't necessarily pinpoint the source of pain. The most reliable way to diagnose z-joint pain is to numb the medial branch nerves and observe the results.

Medial Branch Block (MBB)

Medial branch block, or MBB, is considered the most valid diagnostic test for z-joint pain. As you may recall from Chapter 1, my patient Eric underwent this procedure to help locate the source of his back issues.

During MBB, your physician injects a short-acting anesthetic along the medial branch nerves. Once the medication takes effect, you'll be asked to move in ways that normally hurt your back. Significant pain relief (greater than 80 percent) is considered a good diagnostic indicator of z-joint-related pain.

In most cases, your back pain will return as soon as the anesthetic wears off. However, MBB can occasionally break the cycle of pain and muscle spasm that is causing your discomfort, providing days or even weeks of relief.

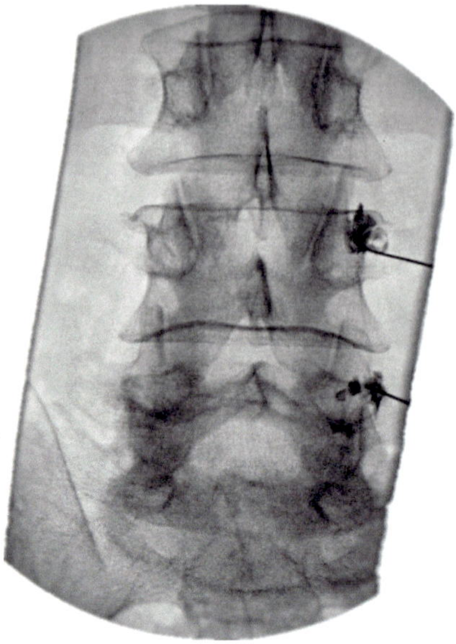

Figure 18: Needles perpendicular to the location of the medial branch nerves. Contrast dye shows verification of proper flow along these nerves prior to injecting local anesthetic for a medial branch block procedure. The patient is a 27-year-old professional athlete.

If the first injection works, your physician should have you return after a week or so to repeat the procedure. This is necessary because a single MBB has a high false positive rate (as high as 40 percent in some studies). During the second injection, the physician may use a different anesthetic that is shorter- or longer-acting than the first. If this "double block" provides relief, it's strong evidence that your pain indeed originates in the z-joint.

Does MBB work?

The strongest evidence for MBB as a diagnostic tool comes from a study by Kaplan and colleagues, which involved a small group of participants with no history of low back pain. The team began the experiment by injecting the z-joint capsules of the subjects with contrast medium until the increased pressure and distention resulted in pain. A week later, researchers split the patients into two groups. The treatment group underwent true MBB while the control group was given a "sham" nerve block. The participants then underwent a second course of capsular distention. All of the patients in the sham therapy group experienced pain—but only one of nine in the MBB group reported any discomfort.

Researchers concluded that when properly administered, MBB was an effective diagnostic indicator of z-joint pain.

Is MBB right for you?

MBB is safe for most patients with suspected z-joint pain that has not responded to three months of conservative treatment. However, talk to your doctor if you are taking blood-thinning medications such as Coumadin or Plavix. In some cases, your physician will recommend stopping your medication for several days so you can safely undergo an MBB. You should not have an MBB if you have signs of spine infection such as fever or a history of IV drug use.

What to expect

Like many other interventional spine procedures, an MBB is performed on an x-ray sensitive table using a fluoroscope to visualize the position of the needle. Your physician will ask you to lie face down, and a nurse or assistant will monitor your heartbeat, blood pressure, and blood oxygen levels. You will receive a small injection to numb the skin and underlying tissue at the puncture site. (While this is usually no more painful than a flu shot, a lot of people say it's the worst part of the procedure.)

Once you're numb, the physician will inject a contrast agent and then an anesthetic along the medial branch nerve of the appropriate z-joint or joints. The entire procedure takes just a few minutes, depending on the number of joints tested and the skill of your doctor. Afterward, you'll be asked to bend, twist, and perform other movements that normally hurt your back. Your doctor will also give you a "pain diary" to take home, where you'll record the intensity and duration of your discomfort over the next several hours. It's very important to fill this out thoroughly and accurately, as your answers will provide important diagnostic information.

Risks and side effects

MBB is generally safe. Afterward, you may notice numbness and mild soreness at the injection site, which usually disappear within a week or so.

After care.

If you were sedated during the procedure, you may feel drowsy and should avoid driving for at least twelve hours. Your doctor may prescribe painkillers to help you cope with the resulting pain and stiffness. Applying cold packs for the first couple of days may further reduce pain and swelling and promote recovery. Resume your normal activities as you feel able. You can usually return to work the next day.

Treatments for Z-Joint Pain

Once your physician has identified and confirmed which z-joints are causing your pain, spinal arthritis can often be treated with a low-risk procedure called radiofrequency neurotomy. Back surgery, which is also appropriate in some cases, is discussed in detail in Chapter 9.

Radiofrequency Neurotomy (RFN)

This minimally invasive treatment uses heat energy to cauterize a small portion of the medial branch nerves. The resulting lesion prevents the transmission of pain signals between the z-joint and spinal cord. (Think of it as a type of branch block that lasts months, not hours.) During the procedure, a tiny electrode—so small it can be inserted through the tip of a needle—is placed parallel to the nerve and heated to a temperature of 85 degrees Celsius (185 degrees Fahrenheit) for ninety seconds. Depending on the probe size used, the resulting lesion is anywhere from five to ten millimeters in diameter. Your physician will usually create multiple lesions to cauterize an adequate volume of nerve tissue.

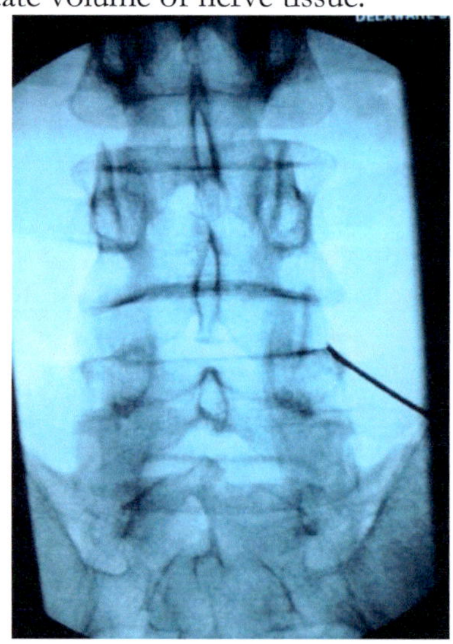

Figure 19: The above patient underwent lumbar radiofrequency neurotomy that provided sustained relief for the next three years. Note that the probe tip is positioned exactly parallel to the medial branch nerve for precise cauterization.

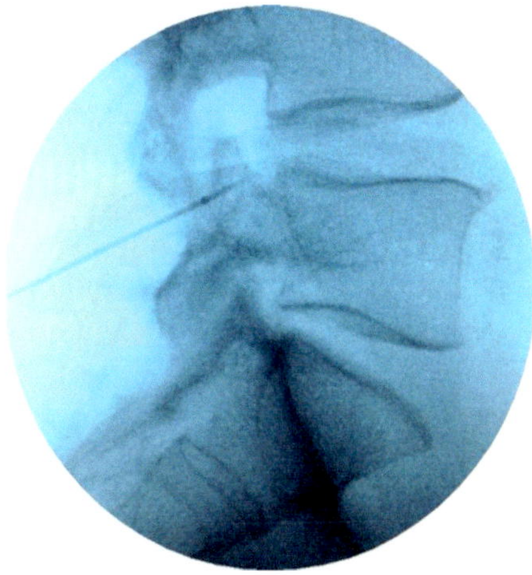

Figure 20: Lateral (side) view of the same radiofrequency probe along the course of the medial branch nerve.

Does RFN work?

Eric in Chapter 1 has undergone several successful RFN procedures that have allowed him to return to his job, sports, and other activities. His pain eventually returns after about twelve months when his nerves regenerate. So far, his response has been positive each time we've repeated the treatment.

Robust evidence suggests that Eric's experience is typical. Researchers at the San Francisco Spine Institute recently conducted a chart review of twenty patients treated with a series of RFNs. After the first procedure, 85 percent of the patients reported a 50 percent or greater reduction in pain intensity. On average, this relief lasted 10.5 months. Results for subsequent procedures were statistically identical.

In recent years, some experts have questioned the effectiveness of RFN. In most cases, they're relying on one of several high-profile studies that unfortunately include serious methodological flaws. In some of these trials, researchers selected participants based on inappropriate diagnostic criteria, such as response to a single medial branch block. (Remember when we discussed the importance of double block MBBs and reproducible relief?) In other trials, physicians performed RFN using techniques shown to be ineffective or inferior (for example, wrong-size needle or improper needle placement). Unfortunately, several of these studies are cited in systematic reviews (including a Cochrane Review), lending them a veneer of legitimacy.

These conclusions were squarely challenged in a 2009 analysis conducted by prominent interventional spine pain researchers Nikolai Bogduk, Paul Dreyfuss, and Jayantilal Govind. Their paper pointed out methodological problems in several oft-quoted studies. They also demonstrated that when these flawed trials are removed from the analysis, there is strong evidence that RFN relieves pain and improves function.

Is RFN right for you?

RFN may be appropriate if your joint pain is confirmed by multiple nerve blocks and hasn't improved after at least three months of conservative therapy. Success is most likely when your response to MBB is significant (at least 80 percent relief after each injection). RFN is possible after back surgery provided the nerve is still accessible. A repeat RFN is appropriate if you've experienced six months or more of relief after past procedures.

What to expect

Although RFN is technically different from a medial branch block, the patient experience is much the same. Your physician will position you face down on an x-ray-sensitive table. Under fluoroscopic guidance, he or she inserts a hollow needle through the skin and positions it parallel to the medial branch nerves. A tiny radiofrequency probe is threaded through this needle to the target nerve. Multiple views are checked to verify correct placement and ensure the lesion won't impact any larger nerves or structures.

Once the probe is positioned in the optimal anatomic location, your doctor injects an anesthetic to numb the medial branch nerve. The heated probe is then applied for about two minutes to create the tiny lesion.

Risks and side effects

After RFN, you may notice increased pain and soreness for three to five days. Other symptoms like itching, burning, and sensitivity can persist for several weeks. Your doctor can prescribe medication to manage these symptoms if they bother you or keep you from your regular activities. Serious complications of RFN, such as nerve injury, are extremely rare.

What should I do after RFN?

Avoid driving for at least twelve hours after the procedure if you received IV sedation. Applying cold packs for the first two days may also help reduce pain and inflammation and promote healing. Your physician may also prescribe painkillers if needed. Return to your normal activities as you feel able, beginning the next day.

Marvin: "These days, I barely think about my back."

Within six weeks, Marvin was pain-free for the first time in years. After a second medial branch block confirmed the location of his joint pain, he underwent lumbar radiofrequency neurotomy and was extremely satisfied with the results.

Marvin can now tolerate two-to-three-hour road trips—and longer ones if he takes frequent breaks. He is now able to accept some longer assignments and no longer worries about losing his job.

After about ten months, Marvin's pain began to increase as his medial branch nerves regenerated. Fortunately, his second course of RFN proved just as effective as the first.

Marvin knows that finding the right doctor is difficult. "I did a lot of reading and educating myself, but my family doctor and pain management doctor pretty much blew off my questions," he says. "It's important to keep looking until you find someone who really listens, talks you through the options, and lets you make the final call."

In addition, he's learned the importance of proper back care. "Now that I'm not in pain, I make sure I do thirty minutes of walking every day, which helps keep the weight off," he says. "I still do the exercises and stretches I learned in physical therapy, and yes, I still do yoga. I even taught it to a few of my trucker buddies."

Key Points

- Z-joint pain is common but difficult to distinguish from other sources of back pain without specialized tests.
- Symptoms may come on gradually and often occur in episodes. Mild cases can be managed with over-the-counter painkillers.
- Once the painful z-joint is verified by a medial branch block,

interventional treatments like radiofrequency ablation may provide significant relief lasting six to twelve months.

Your z-joints aren't the only joints in your back subject to painful flare-ups. In the next chapter we'll discuss the sacroiliac joints, another common generator of low back pain.

6

SACROILIAC JOINT PAIN: A REAL PAIN IN THE BUTT

When John, a busy dad of two, was diagnosed with amyotrophic lateral sclerosis (ALS) at age fifty, he decided to make every moment count. "After the shock wore off, I realized I had choices," he says. "I could mope around and wait for the paralysis to overtake me. Or I could get busy on my bucket list."

John set out to do the latter. He booked tables at his favorite restaurants and whisked his two teenagers off for a deep sea fishing holiday. And because the idea had always intrigued him, he signed himself and the missus up for ballroom dancing lessons. His life was as full as it had ever been. Only one thing held him back.

Five years ago, John was sipping a beer on a friend's patio when he accidentally stepped off the edge, lost his balance, and fell. He landed hard on his bottom, and ever since he'd been plagued by nagging pain in his left hip. His family doctor referred him to an excellent physiatrist, who diagnosed him with sacroiliac joint pain. Anesthetic injections provided temporary relief, but eventually the pain came back.

In 2012, John experienced his worst flare-up ever. The pain was constant and so intense it woke him several times a night. He couldn't seem to get into a comfortable position, and the slightest sneeze or cough sent a jolt of agony through his torso. Walking and driving were so painful that he couldn't bear more than ten minutes of either. Even sitting through a movie was torture.

John's physiatrist suggested that his ALS, which was by now impacting his core and pelvic muscles, might be increasing the strain on his back. At her recommendation, he tried physical therapy and spinal manipulation, but nothing seemed to help.

At his next appointment, John broke down and shared his growing anxiety and depression. "I was afraid this was the beginning of the end," he says. "I was going to be sick and drugged up for the rest of my life." Fortunately, his physiatrist was familiar with interventional spine procedures and explained the many treatment options available. She referred John to our center, where a diagnostic workup confirmed his sacroiliac joint as the probable source of his pain.

Sacroiliac Joint Pain: What Is It?

Sacroiliac (SI) joint pain like John's has been reported by various researchers to account for 15 to 25 percent of chronic low back pain cases. However, most of these studies didn't first rule out other common pain sources like the discs and z-joints that refer to the sacroiliac region. What's more, SI joint pain doesn't necessarily stand alone—it coexists with other painful back conditions more than 35 percent of the time. (Which brings up an important point: while this book focuses on one problem at a time, it's quite common to have more than one thing wrong with you.)

Your two SI joints are complex systems of bone, cartilage, and ligaments that connect the base of your spine to your hipbones on either side. Like the z-joints, they're enclosed in fluid-filled capsules. A system of strong ligaments holds the joints together and limits their rotation to about two degrees. These ligaments also serve as attachment points for the large muscles in your buttocks and thighs that stabilize the pelvis and lend further strength to the SI joint.

Provocative studies (those that use injections or probing to cause sensation) have shown that the SI joints contain pain-sensing nociceptors in both joint capsules and the surrounding ligaments. Most of these nerve endings derive from the lateral branch nerves, which exit the sacrum bone through holes called foramina and enter the joint from behind. In most people, the L5 dorsal ramus (spinal nerve branch extending backward from that level) contributes some innervation as well. The depth, number, and location of these nerves are a little different in every person

Though we'll focus on the nerves of the posterior (back side) of the SI joint, it's important to note that some nerves also enter from the front as well. At present, no procedure is available that can block these anterior (front side) nerves. For this reason, it's sometimes difficult to completely eliminate SI joint pain, though the level of discomfort can often be reduced.

What Causes SI Joint Pain?

Sacroiliac joint pain often arises due to mechanical problems in one or both joints. Sometimes a joint gets "stuck" and doesn't move smoothly around the hipbone. The other joint typically compensates by working harder and through a greater range of motion. Over time, this extra strain can result in pain.

Trauma is another common trigger. A torn ligament can cause the bony surfaces of the sacrum and ileum (which are ridged and grooved respectively for maximum stability) to misalign. The resultant "grinding" tears and irritates the joint cartilage, which eventually leads to pain and inflammation. Additionally, some experts have theorized that hormonal changes during pregnancy can also loosen the ligaments. This allows the extra joint movement to accommodate childbirth.

Like the z-joints, the SI joints can develop painful arthritis that limits range of motion. This may be due to natural age changes or an inflammatory disease like lupus or psoriasis.

Finally, pain in your sacroiliac area can occur even when the joint itself is functioning normally. Many spinal conditions can actually send or "refer" pain to the sacroiliac area, including problems of the z-joints, intervertebral discs, and spinal nerves.

What Are the Symptoms?

SI joint pain usually (but not always) occurs on just one side of the back. It can also radiate to the buttock, hamstring, or groin on the same side of the body. Some patients notice popping or clicking in the pelvic area during certain movements. One leg may feel weaker or less stable than the other.

Who's at Risk?

Age is a major risk factor for SI joint problems. In addition, people with light builds tend to have lower bone densities and are therefore at greater risk for arthritis, bone spurs, and fractures as they get older.

Like John, about half of all people diagnosed with SI joint dysfunction have a history of trauma. Common causes include falls, motor vehicle accidents, and cumulative stresses like heavy lifting.

Spinal fusion surgery appears to increase the risk of SI joint problems down the road. Computer modeling suggests that fusion increases both motion and stress within the SI joint. Studies have found that about 40 percent of surgical patients who continue to have chronic back pain have SI joint involvement. (For more information, see Chapter 10 on failed back surgery syndrome.)

As noted above, SI joint pain is common in pregnant women and new mothers. One theory is that the body releases certain hormones that open the joints to facilitate childbirth. During pregnancy, changes in gait and weight gain may also increase stress on the sacroiliac area.

Diagnosis

Diagnosing SI joint pain is often difficult due to the multiple nerves and joint structures involved. Furthermore, because everyone's SI joints are "wired" differently, the condition produces a wide variety of pain patterns. Imaging studies like bone scans and CT scans often miss important diagnostic clues. For these reasons, most experts agree that the best diagnostic procedure is a double block (two anesthetic injections) of the lateral branch nerves that transmit pain signals between the joint and the spinal cord.

To confidently diagnose sacroiliac joint pain, your physician may need to rule out other common problems like internal disc disruption syndrome and z-joint pain, both of which sometimes "send" pain to the sacroiliac region. Diagnostic procedures for these conditions are discussed in Chapters 4 and 5 respectively.

Physical Examination and Stress Maneuvers

No single physical exam finding or test has been shown to reliably diagnose SI joint pain. However, studies suggest that certain combinations of stress maneuvers—tests which involve bending, pressing, and pulling of the legs and hips—can often differentiate SI joint problems from other types of back pain. A 2003 Australian study found that a positive (painful) response to three out of the following tests was a strong diagnostic indicator:

- **Gaenslen's test**. The doctor will have you pull one knee to your chest while allowing the other to drop over the edge of the exam table. This stresses both SI joints simultaneously.
- **Thigh thrust**. Your doctor flexes your hip at a 90-degree angle,

bends your knee, and presses downward on the knee to create shearing force on the SI joint.

- **Sacral thrust**. Your doctor presses directly on your sacrum area as you lie on your stomach.
- **Compression**. While you lie on one side, your physician presses downward on your hip to open the SI joint.
- **Distraction**. While you lie on your back, the examiner presses the front sides of your SI joints to open them.

Lateral Branch Block

While a physical exam can provide important clues, a lateral branch block helps your doctor to diagnose SI joint problems with confidence. To perform this test, your physician injects a mixture of anesthetic and contrast agent near the nerves of your low back that connect your SI joint and spinal cord. LBB is considered positive if you experience at least 80 percent reduction in pain intensity when twisting or bending in ways that normally hurt your back. The pain must also return as the anesthetic wears off. Provided there are no tears to allow for anesthetic leakage, other clinicians make the diagnosis by instilling local anesthetic into the joint itself.

Like all procedures, LBB has limitations. Research suggests that single injections have a relatively high false positive rate—as high as 48 percent in one study. And while LBB can generally detect ligament pain, it's less reliable for pinpointing problems within the joint capsule itself. A rigorous controlled study by Dreyfuss, Bogduk, and colleagues found that LBB correctly diagnosed SI joint pain in 70 percent of patients when multiple injections were delivered at different sites and depths. The International Spine Intervention Society therefore recommends that patients undergo a second block to confirm the findings of the first before a firm diagnosis is made.

The patient experience, risks, side effects, and aftercare considerations for LBB are very similar to those for medial branch block, which is discussed in detail in Chapter 5.

Treatment

If you're diagnosed with SI joint pain, your doctor may recommend any number of treatment approaches, including conservative therapy, steroid injections, interventional procedures, or surgery.

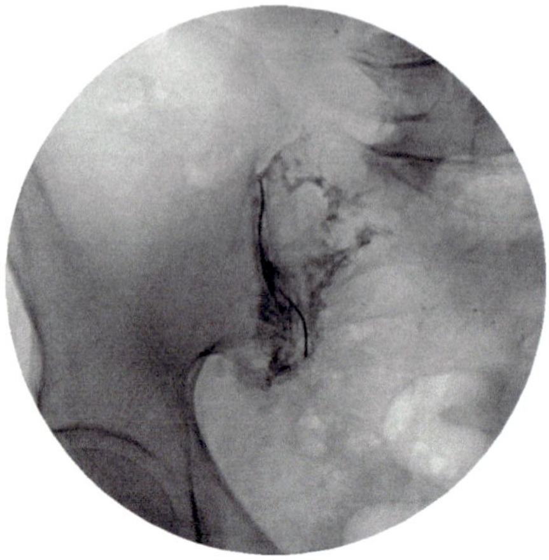

Figure 21: Spinal needle within the left sacroiliac joint. Contrast material in the joint (arthrogram) shows its shape as well as some diverticuli (outpouching pockets of the joint capsule). This patient had left buttock pain with non-diagnostic spinal nerve blocks, non-diagnostic z-joint blocks, and non-diagnostic disc stimulation. He ultimately underwent an extremely successful radiofrequency neurotomy of his sacroiliac joint.

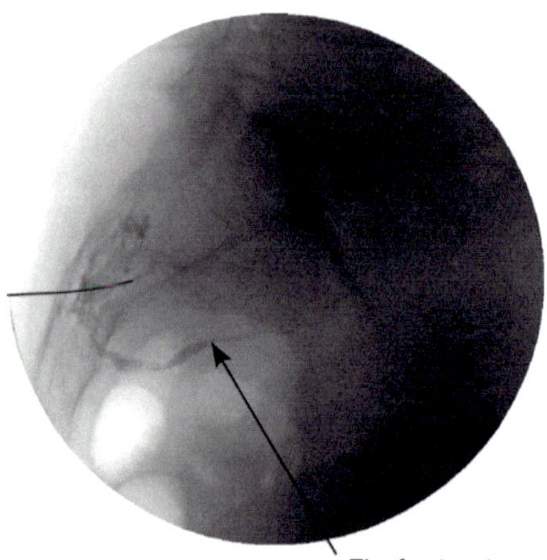

Figure 22: Side view of the same procedure. Notice the needle in the joint. The contrast is contained within the capsule, indicating that it is intact. Capsule tears are common and often painless.

Lateral Branch Neurotomy

In Chapters 4 and 5, we discussed radiofrequency neurotomy, a minimally invasive denervation procedure used to treat z-joint pain. The mechanics of lateral branch neurotomy are much the same. A probe is inserted parallel to the target nerve under fluoroscopic guidance and heated to about 85 degrees Celsius for ninety seconds to create a lesion. This prevents the nerve from transmitting pain signals from the SI joint to the spinal cord, resulting in partial or complete relief.

Because the SI joints are innervated by multiple nerves (the structure and location of which vary from person to person), your doctor will generally create several lesions to ensure that a sufficient volume of tissue is cauterized. In some cases, an internally cooled probe is used to create larger lesions (about 10 millimeters across versus 5 with traditional probes). Use of a cold probe also prevents scorching of the surrounding tissue, which tends to reduce the amount of pain you feel in the days following the procedure.

Does lateral branch neurotomy work?

LBN is relatively new and somewhat controversial among physicians. While studies generally support its efficacy in carefully selected patients (with about two-thirds experiencing significant relief), there's still a lot of research to be done.

In a 2013 Austrian study, researchers reviewed the cases of one hundred twenty-six patients treated by cooled-probe lateral branch neurotomy. All had chronic low back pain with SI joint involvement confirmed by nerve block injection. At four to six weeks follow-up:

- 86 percent of participants were still experiencing significant pain relief.
- 96 percent reported improved quality of life.
- 100 percent of the narcotic users in the group had stopped or reduced their intake.

As with other denervation procedures, the benefits of lateral branch neurotomy wear off as the nerve regenerates. However, at one year follow-up:

- 48 percent of the subjects were still experiencing significant pain relief.
- 85 percent still reported improved quality of life.
- 67 percent were still taking no or fewer narcotics than before the procedure.

The team continued to follow the subjects and found that some experienced significant benefits for twenty months or longer. They noted that these results are generally consistent with past trials of lateral and medial branch neurotomy.

Is lateral branch neurotomy right for you?

LBN is generally appropriate for people with chronic low back pain (greater than three months in duration) when SI joint involvement has been confirmed by a double lateral branch block and referred pain sources have been ruled out. Relief should be reproducible when the block is repeated at different sites, depths, and with different anesthetics.

What to expect

The patient experience, risk factors, side effects, and aftercare considerations for LBN are very similar to those of medial branch neurotomy, which is discussed in depth in Chapter 5.

Other Interventional Treatments

Lesioning of the nerves within the joint capsule appears to be an effective approach in about one-third of patients with confirmed SI joint pain. While this denervates only the back third of the joint, it may be a good alternative for people with arthritis and other intra-joint conditions. A 2001 trial of this procedure produced significant relief in twelve of thirty-three patients. Additional research is needed to help doctors identify those most likely to benefit.

John: Making Each Day Count

Since he arrived at our center, John has made excellent progress. During his diagnostic work-up, he underwent a lateral branch block that seemed to have a positive effect not only on his SI joint but also on his weakened pelvic muscles. Afterward, he was able to stand and walk without pain, and these benefits actually persisted for about three months after the procedure. He even felt well enough during this period to take a four-hour flight to California and visit with his parents.

John ultimately underwent radiofrequency neurotomy of the nerves within his SI joint capsule. One year later, he's still pain free. He's able to stand and walk for extended periods and is even talking about resuming his ballroom lessons. Best of all, he's enjoying every moment with friends and family. "It's really been an incredible time for me," he says. "I did so well at checking off my bucket list, I actually had to add a few things."

Key Points

- SI joint pain usually affects one side of the back and may radiate to the buttocks, groin, or hamstring.
- The most common causes of SI joint pain involve mechanical problems of the bones and ligaments.
- Painful conditions elsewhere in the back can sometimes transmit their pain to the SI joint. These "referred" pain sources must be ruled out for a firm diagnosis of SI joint pain.
- The most accurate diagnostic test for SI joint pain is a double lateral branch block.
- Evidence suggests that denervation via radiofrequency neurotomy can relieve SI joint pain in the majority of carefully selected patients.

So far in this handbook, we've focused on mechanical causes of back pain. But what about when the source of the pain is the nerve itself? Next, we'll look at two common causes of nerve pain: disc herniation (Chapter 7) and spinal stenosis (Chapter 8).

7

DISC HERNIATION RADICULAR PAIN: WHEN DISCS GET ON YOUR NERVES

Cliff had been an avid distance runner since high school, but was never competitive in the sport until he turned fifty. Suddenly he was officially a "master" and placing consistently in his new age category. "It was like getting a second wind," he recalls. "I'd been thinking about cutting back my running and playing more golf, because I felt like I needed a more social hobby. But as soon as I started winning, I was hooked."

Cliff ramped up his training and began traveling to marathons in neighboring states. He also set his sights on a new goal—the Leadville 100 ultra marathon in Colorado. His two teenage daughters were thrilled and took turns circling the park with him each Sunday. But as his training runs lengthened beyond fifty miles, a new obstacle surfaced—a persistent pain in the right side of his groin.

His family doctor insisted it was a muscle pull that would go away on its own. Instead, it got worse. Within a few months, the ache was constant and keeping him awake at night. Cliff scrapped his plans for Leadville, cut back his training, and enrolled in intensive physical therapy. He was motivated and very serious about getting better, yet the pain kept plaguing him.

Over the next three years, Cliff saw four physical therapists and more specialists than he could count. He still ran as much as he could, but usually no more than a few miles a week. When his wife convinced him to enter a 5K with her, he barely finished. "Eighty-year-olds and people with giant strollers were blowing right past me," he recalls. "It was beyond depressing."

Pain, disappointment, and sleep deprivation were all taking a toll on his family. His daughters, who had been so supportive of his running, now seemed to avoid him. When his wife tried to talk to him about his "anger issues," he stormed out of the house. By the weekend, he was far too miserable to hit the golf course with his friends. "It seemed like my life was over," he says. "I started to feel really hopeless about the future."

Cliff came to our center for what he called his "thirteenth opinion." Like many of our patients, he showed up with an armload of x-rays, reports, and other documentation, all of which pointed to a herniated L2/3 intervertebral disc.

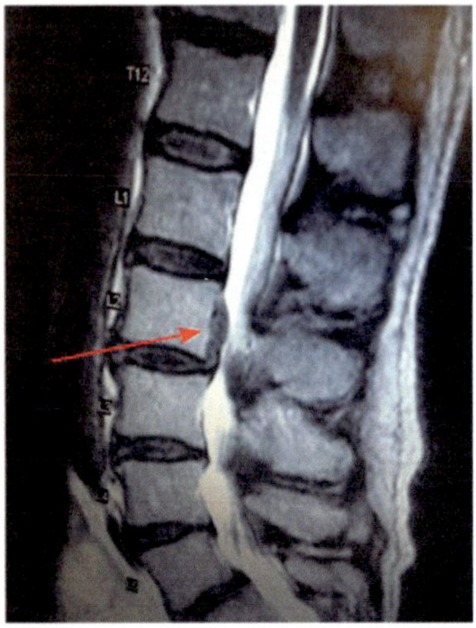

Figure 23: Lateral side view of Cliff's L2/3 extrusion running up the back side of the L2 vertebral body on the left.

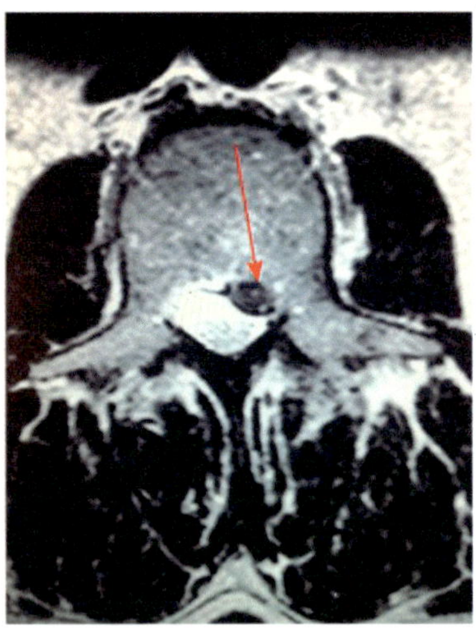

Figure 24: Cliff's axial cross section MRI: The arrows depict a left-sided disc extrusion herniation running up behind the L2 intervertebral body.

"Would epidurals help?" Cliff asked when I showed him the film.

I explained that with his type of disc herniation, they were not usually successful on a long-term basis. Then I gave him a couple of epidural steroid injections at the L3 level. Afterward, he was able to jog down the hall without pain for the first time in nearly a year.

Disc Herniation Radicular Pain: What Is It?

Disc herniation pain is relatively common, occurring in about 1 to 3 percent of the population at any given time. However, patients and physicians often mistake the resulting back and leg pain for a sprain, muscle strain, or even peripheral artery disease. Fortunately, most cases resolve on their own within a month or two. But for patients who go on to have chronic pain, there can be long delays in treatment due to misdiagnoses and poor understanding of the condition among medical professionals.

Disc Changes

A bulging disc like Cliff's often causes radicular (radiating) pain that follows the path of the spinal nerves into the lower limbs. As you may recall from Chapter 4, the intervertebral discs that connect and cushion the bones of the spine are prone to internal tears that radiate outward from the center like the spokes of a wheel. Herniation occurs when the gel-like inner nucleus of the disc (called the nucleus pulposus) spreads along these tears, causing the disc to bulge. If the rupture extends to the disc surface, the nucleus may even balloon outward through the opening.

Disc herniation occurs along a spectrum of severity listed here from least to most serious:

- **Bulge**. Generalized extension of the disc due to breakdown of the annular wall.
- **Protrusion**. Localized outpouching of the annulus causes a "bump" to form on the disc surface.
- **Extrusion**. Nucleus pulposus material hangs out of a tear in the annulus
- **Sequestration**. A piece of the nucleus pulposus breaks off into the epidural space.

Nerve Compression

Herniation is most common at the rear of the disc where mechanical pressures are greatest. Unfortunately, this is also the area where the nerve roots split off from the spinal cord, exiting the spinal column through side portals called foramina. At each level of the spine, associated nerve roots coalesce into a bud called the ganglion to form a spinal nerve.

As we discussed in Chapter 4, disc tears can provoke certain chemical reactions, which are interpreted by sensory nerve endings as pain. In the case of herniation, bulging discs can cause additional discomfort by pressing on the nerve roots or ganglia. This results in radicular (radiating) pain that extends along the affected nerve to the buttocks, legs, and feet. The pain may be continuous along the length of the nerve or occur in patches. Discomfort is typically felt in the skin area, or dermatome, whose nerve endings derive from the affected nerve root.

Spinal nerve dysfunction due to compression or irritation is called "radiculopathy." Signs include muscle weakness and diminished reflexes. The person may also loose the ability to sense some stimuli (light touch, pinpricks) in the affected area.

Chemical Irritation

There is evidence that herniation can cause pain even when the bulging disc doesn't compress the nerves. The nucleus pulposus is composed of algogens—substances that irritate and increase the sensitivity of nerve tissue. Research suggests that contact with an extruded nucleus may provoke an inflammatory response in nearby nerve roots, resulting in intense pain.

This condition, known as chemical radiculitis, has been successfully modeled in rats. In a 2012 study, researchers harvested nucleus pulposus cells from the animals, then re-injected these into the rats' epidural spaces to simulate disc extrusion. Introduction of nuclear material provoked a measurable inflammatory response, causing an elevation in chemicals called cytokines that typically accompanies injury. This response strongly suggests that chemical changes play a key role in radicular pain.

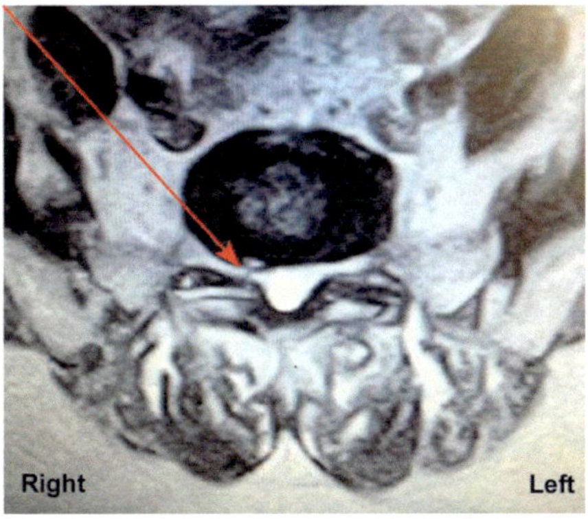

Figure 25: Right lateral recess protrusion with high intensity bright signal in the outer layer of the herniation where the right L5 spinal nerve traverses behind the L4/5 disc

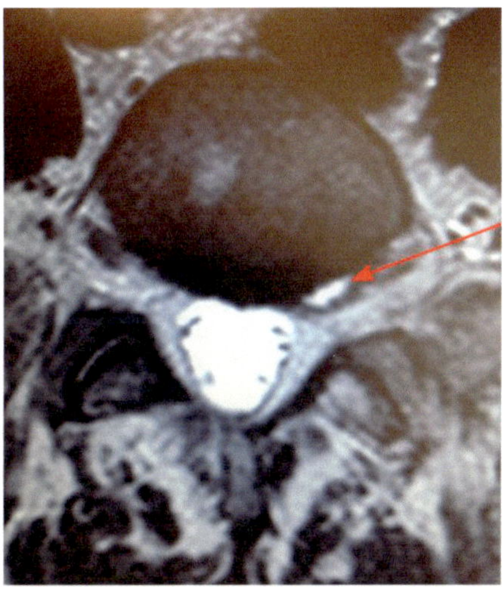

Figure 26: Cross-sectional view of the L5/1 disc showing a high-intensity zone bright white signal at the level of the left L5 nerve consistent with chemical radiculitis. The patient was a 37-year-old woman with severe pain in her lower back and left outer calf. Left L5 transforaminal epidural steroid injections resolved her leg pain.

What Are the Symptoms of Disc Herniation?

Disc herniation often causes low back pain that radiates to the buttocks and lower limbs. Pain may be sharp, burning, or tingly—sensations often associated with nerve pain. However, the discomfort may also be dull or achy like that of a sprain or bruise. Some patients also notice muscle weakness in the legs, which may present as clumsiness, falling, or changes in gait.

Certain activities or postures may shift the bulging disc so that it puts additional pressure on the nerve. Pain may worsen when walking (especially if the herniation is in the foramen) or sitting for extended periods (when the disc protrudes into the central canal).

Radicular leg pain is often mistaken for other conditions, including peripheral artery disease, muscle and tendon sprains, hip arthritis, peripheral nerve problems, or bursitis. It can also mimic sacroiliac joint pain, another common pain generator.

Diagnosis

In order to treat disc herniation, your physician must first identify the affected nerve roots and to rule out other painful conditions. This is usually accomplished over several visits through a combination of imaging, history, and physical examination.

Imaging

Three-dimensional imaging modalities like MRI and CT are frequently used as a starting point for planning an effective diagnostic examination. These tests detect bumps or bulges along the disc surface. However, even when evident, these features may not necessarily be the source of the pain. A knowledgeable spine physician will continue searching for evidence before making a firm diagnosis.

Patient History

Every spinal level is associated with a spinal nerve formed from its associated nerve roots. Nerves originating at each level carry sensory and motor signals to a different part of the body. These regions can be mapped on the skin as dermatomes. Pain within a dermatome can signal a problem with the nerve root that governs it.

To uncover clues about the source of your pain, your doctor may have you complete a "pain drawing." While not a definitive diagnostic tool, this map can uncover interesting patterns. Pain that occurs in several areas of the same dermatome (parts of the buttock, thigh, and foot, for example) might suggest nerve root involvement. Also, a significant number of patients whose back pain radiates below the knee are later diagnosed with disc herniation.

Pain mapping has its limits. Radicular pain may be felt uniformly across the dermatome or just in certain parts. Some dermatomes (L4 and L5, for example) occur in long, narrow bands that run parallel along the length of the leg, making it difficult to locate the pain precisely. Dermatomes may overlap by as much as 50 percent in some parts of the body. And finally, many people are just "wired" differently— skin innervated by L5 in one person may be associated with S1 in another. Hence, while they provide a starting point, pain maps need to be interpreted alongside other diagnostic information.

Neurologic Exam

Up to 80 percent of patients with radicular pain also experience some neurologic changes. A careful neurologic exam can provide clues as to the level of the lesion. It can also uncover related problems such as a pinched or diseased peripheral nerve within the leg.

Sensory testing involves probing of the dermatomes with light pressure, hard pressure, pinpricks, and vibrations—each of which stimulates a different type of nerve fiber. Your physician will ask you to indicate when you feel pain, tingling, burning, numbness, or any other unusual sensation. If multiple skin areas within the same dermatome show sensory changes, this could indicate a problem with the associated nerve root.

Muscle weakness may result when a disc compresses the motor portion of a nerve. People with radiculopathy sometimes report changes in their gait or balance, but often these changes are so subtle that they go unnoticed. During the neurologic exam, your physician will have you perform certain maneuvers that test your muscle strength. Because most muscles are innervated by nerve roots from two adjacent levels, patterns of weakness may provide clues as to the location of the problem. For example, if a weak muscle is innervated by L1/2 and L2/3, this could indicate a problem with the nerve roots at L2. However, your lack of strength could also be due to deconditioning, joint problems, or the fact that the leg being tested is throbbing in pain.

Finally, your physician will test reflex points in your legs and feet. Reflexes are involuntary reactions to certain stimuli (a touch, a tap) that are controlled by your spinal cord. Reflexes in your knees and ankles may weaken or even disappear when a motor nerve is compressed.

Orthopedic Exam

Movements which increase pressure on the lumbar spinal nerves are quite useful in diagnosing disc herniation. The maneuver best supported by research is the crossed straight leg raise (SLR). The patient lies face up and slowly raises the affected leg while letting the other leg drop over the edge of the exam table. If pain occurs while the raised leg is at a low angle (less than seventy degrees), nerve compression is very likely present. In fact, studies have demonstrated that a painful SLR is predictive of disc herniation over 90 percent of the time.

On the other hand, a negative result doesn't rule out radiculopathy. The SLR and similar maneuvers are less sensitive in older patients and for disc herniation at higher spine levels. Nor can physical tests detect pain that is due purely to nerve irritation (chemical radiculitis).

Even when a physical test is positive, it still can't tell us what level of the spine is affected. That's one reason that corroborating evidence (imaging studies, pain patterns, and sensory data) is so important in formulating a diagnosis.

Spinal Nerve Block

This test has shown great promise in its ability to identify a specific spinal nerve root as the pain source. As in other "block" studies, the physician injects a small amount of anesthetic into the sheath of the target nerve under fluoroscopic guidance. The patient is then asked to move in ways that usually provoke pain and report the results. Reproduction of your normal pain during injection followed by significant relief under anesthetic signals nerve involvement at the injected level.

A recent study of patients who underwent spinal nerve block and later had back surgery found that the procedure diagnosed radicular pain associated with disc herniation correctly in eighteen of nineteen cases. By comparison, CT scans detected signs in only fourteen.

Because it's possible to injure the spinal nerve during the block procedure, it's imperative that a physician with considerable skill and extensive, supervised training perform the procedure. Afterward, about 10 percent of patients have side effects such as a temporary increase in pain, headache, nausea, increased blood sugar, fainting, and flushed face. These almost always resolve within a few days.

Treatments

Treatment for disc herniation radicular pain may consist of steroid injections, percutaneous decompression, or surgery. The remainder of this chapter focuses on minimally invasive approaches. Surgery is discussed in detail in Chapter 9.

Epidural Steroid Injections

As you may recall from Chapter 4, steroid injections have been used as a somewhat controversial treatment for internal disc disruption syndrome. In the case of disc herniation, the physician injects a dose of strong anti-inflammatory medication along the spinal nerve through the foramen. For maximum safety and accuracy, this is always performed under x-ray guidance. In the old days, it was done blindly. The physician would estimate the location and angle of approach and insert the needle. If the patient experienced leg pain during the injection, the needle was presumed to be in the right spot. Thanks to technological advances, the process is now far safer—not to mention more pleasant for the patient.

When effective, steroid injections relieve pain and reduce swelling, sensitivity, and irritation around the nerve. In some people, these benefits gradually wear off over a period of months. However, the procedure can be repeated as needed to keep the pain at bay.

The evidence supporting epidural steroid injections as a treatment for disc herniation radicular pain is much stronger than for other back problems. In a 2013 systematic review of thirty-nine studies, researchers concluded that while transforaminal steroid injection was not universally effective, it benefited a significant number of patients. About 60 percent of study participants achieved 50 percent or greater pain relief for one to two months. For 40 percent of patients, the relief lasted at least a year. In addition, participants showed significant gains in functional ability and were less likely to undergo surgery later. Researchers noted that steroid injections were most effective for patients with contained herniation that caused minimal nerve compression.

Patient experience, side effects and aftercare considerations for transforaminal steroid injections are discussed in detail in Chapter 4.

Percutaneous Decompression

Some treatments for disc herniation seek to relieve pain by decreasing pressure on the affected nerve root. In the case of surgery, this involves removing all or part of the problematic disc. However, as we'll discuss in Chapter 9, surgery isn't the answer for everyone. Due to the health risks and long recovery times involved, some people opt to try minimally invasive approaches first.

Over the past forty years, researchers have experimented with a number of interventional techniques to treat disc herniation pain. Many of these use lasers, radiofrequency, or chemicals to decrease pressure within the disc. In theory, this reduces the size of bulges and protrusions, which encourages extruded nuclei to slip back inside the disc. Collectively, these techniques are known as percutaneous (through-the-skin) decompression.

Unfortunately, no form of percutaneous depression has proven effective in controlled, randomized trials. Due to the difficulty of controlling for variables like herniation severity and physician skill, very few high-quality studies exist. Based on this limited evidence, percutaneous decompression does appear to be somewhat more successful in people with contained herniation.

Percutaneous decompression may be an alternative to surgery if you have a contained (or partially contained) disc herniation confirmed by spinal imaging. Results appear to be best when pain is radicular and the disc is relatively healthy (in other words, maintaining at least half its normal height).

Cliff: On the Run Again

Epidural steroid injections provided Cliff with several months of relief that allowed him to get his life back on track. His mood improved dramatically when he was able to sleep through the night, and his relationships with his wife and daughters improved. Soon he was back to running, golfing and enjoying an active lifestyle.

As a more permanent solution, Cliff chose to have discectomy surgery that removed a protrusion and relieved the pressure on the nearby nerves. His results were excellent, and within twelve weeks, he was back in training for Leadville (which he hopes to tackle in summer 2013). He's thrilled with the treatment he received and his new lease on life. "If I'd given up on getting better, I'd be a mess today," he says. "I'm glad I went in for my 'thirteenth opinion.'"

Key Points

- Disc herniation occurs when a bulging disc presses against the surrounding nerve roots. The resulting pain and neurological symptoms are often mistaken for other injuries and health problems.
- In some cases of herniation, the nucleus pulposus actually bulges through a crack in the annulus. This can cause chemical irritation of the nerve roots even when no compression is present.
- A disc herniation diagnosis requires a careful combination of history, physical examination, imaging and interventional procedures. Other possible pain sources should be ruled out as well.
- Though treatment usually requires surgery, the condition can often be managed with epidural steroid injections.
- Percutaneous decompression treatments are not well supported by evidence, but may be tried as an alternative to surgery.

In the next chapter we'll discuss yet another cause of nerve pain: spinal stenosis. It involves narrowing of the spinal canal and is especially common in older people.

8

SPINAL STENOSIS RADICULAR PAIN: THE BIG SQUEEZE

Benita, an ICU nurse at a large metropolitan hospital, can still remember the day her waking nightmare began. She and a colleague were transferring an unconscious patient onto a gurney so he could be taken downstairs for x-rays. Normally, they would have used the overhead lift, but they were in a rush and decided hefting him themselves would be less of a hassle. "Boy was I wrong," Benita says. "That was the start of years of doctors, hospitals, tests, and unrelenting pain."

As she lifted the patient, Benita felt nothing unusual. But later that day, she noticed nagging discomfort in her lower back and left hamstring. Over the next few weeks, the dull pain came and went, along with tingling and numbness that made standing and walking uncomfortable. She tried wearing a back brace at work and was fitted with orthopedic shoes. Nothing helped. The pain kept getting worse.

A year later, Benita, sixty-one, could hardly walk and was on disability leave from her nursing job. "These things happen when you get older," her family doctor told her. He insisted that she just needed a few more months of physical therapy. By this point, she was also in pain management and taking narcotic medications daily.

Frustrated, Benita sought a second opinion from an orthopedic specialist. After weeks of testing, she was diagnosed with degenerative disc disease. The doctor said surgery might help, but suggested they try epidural steroid injections first.

The injections worked for almost a year. Benita went back to work. That summer, her garden, which had withered over the previous year, was filled with flowers and vegetables. But then the injections stopped working, and the pain returned with a vengeance.

Six months later, Benita hit a new low. The simple act of standing sent agonizing pain shooting down her leg. She was out of work again, and during her worst days, she used a walker to get around. Her partner Raul, who worked full-time, had to hire a home health nurse to help Benita out of bed in the morning. Morphine provided some fleeting relief, but she hated taking it and would hold off until she was in agony. "I didn't want to spend the rest of my life on dope," she explains.

After enduring four years of pain and disability, Benita cashed out her IRA and traveled to California to undergo an experimental laser procedure. She was elated when she experienced real relief—and devastated when the pain returned just two months later. Raul, worried about Benita's emotional state and her growing dependency on morphine, began scouring the Internet for other options. His search led Benita to our center.

While Benita's discs and z-joints showed degeneration on imaging studies, we were most concerned about the thickening of her spinal ligaments. Cross-sectional MRI imaging showed significant narrowing of her spinal canal, which was most severe at the L4/5 level. An epidural steroid injection provided partial relief, allowing her to walk the length of the hall without assistance. All of these signs pointed to a condition called spinal stenosis as the true source of her pain.

Spinal Stenosis: What Is It?

When a radiologist's report indicates spinal stenosis, it means that parts of the spinal canal appear to be too narrow. In the low back, this can cause compression of the lower spinal cord and nerve roots. It can also restrict the blood supply of individual spinal nerves. The condition may also impact the cauda equina, a bundle of nerves that descend from the base of the spinal cord to innervate the lower limbs.

Spinal stenosis is the most common spine disorder in older people. As we age, our spinal canals naturally narrow due to wear and tear on the intervertebral discs, z-joints, and ligaments. These changes don't necessarily cause symptoms. However, about five out of every thousand people over fifty experience significant discomfort due to compression of the spinal nerves. Leg or hip pain due to spinal stenosis is by far the most common reason for back surgery among people over sixty-five.

Symptomatic spinal stenosis currently impacts between 250,000 and 500,000 Americans, and this number is expected to rise in coming decades due to growth of the elderly population. However, despite the increasing demand for care, the disorder remains poorly understood. At the time of this writing, there is no diagnostic "gold standard" and relatively little scientific evidence to guide treatment decisions. As in Benita's case, this can result in delay of care and the loss of productive life years.

Many physicians still see surgery as a front line treatment for spinal stenosis, but this can be a risky approach in older patients with multiple chronic health conditions. Fortunately, several less invasive treatments for this disorder are showing promise.

What Are the Symptoms of Spinal Stenosis?

The most common sign of spinal stenosis is neurogenic claudication—cramping pain and weakness in the legs that commonly affects the calf, thigh, and buttock. Standing and walking all tend to aggravate the leg pain. However, the discomfort often eases when the person bends forward (for example, when leaning on a walker or pushing a shopping cart) or when sitting. Symptoms may be present in one or both legs.

Spinal stenosis pain is sometimes mistaken for peripheral artery disease (PAD), which also causes leg pain during physical activity. However, PAD pain usually goes away with rest while neurogenic claudication may not.

In addition to claudication, spinal stenosis can cause radicular pain similar to that of a herniated disc. Pain, numbness, or tingling usually radiate from the lower back down the back of the leg. Often, this pain extends below the knee to the calf or foot. Discomfort is typically (but not always) limited to a single dermatome—the area of skin innervated by the affected nerve root.

Other symptoms of spinal stenosis include:

- Back pain (though this is usually less significant than leg pain)
- Muscle weakness
- Diminished reflexes in the knees and ankles

In rare cases, spinal stenosis can result in cauda equina syndrome, a life-threatening impingement of the large nerves that descend from the spinal cord to innervate the organs of the lower abdomen. Seek medical attention immediately if your pain is accompanied by loss of bowel or bladder control. Emergency surgery may be required to correct the problem.

Over time, spinal stenosis pain and disability can cause significant psychosocial problems, including depression, isolation, and sleep difficulties. These secondary symptoms are associated with poorer outcomes. It's therefore important to explore alternative treatments when pain persists.

What Causes Spinal Stenosis?

Spinal stenosis usually overlaps with other spine and joint conditions. For example, a person with stenosis leg pain may also experience mechanical back pain from z-joint arthritis or internal disc disruption syndrome. Conditions such as herniated disc, sacroiliac joint dysfunction, and even hip joint arthritis may contribute to the leg pain felt by stenosis patients. All of these conditions must be properly diagnosed and treated for the best possible outcome.

Degenerative Spine Changes

Spinal stenosis usually arises from degenerative changes to the z-joints, discs, and ligaments. Over time, wear and tear causes thickening of the ligamenta flava, the strong ligaments which connect the vertebral bodies and form part of the spinal canal's wall. Bone spurs (a common result of z-joint arthritis) can also take up room in the canal, as can herniated intervertebral discs. Age-related thinning of the discs sometimes causes the neural foramina to shift, resulting in pinching or compression of the associated nerve roots.

Degenerative Spondylolisthesis

In some cases, degenerative spine changes cause spondylolisthesis, or "spine slippage." This occurs when a vertebral level shifts forward relative to the one below (usually between L4 and L5), narrowing the spinal canal and compressing nearby nerve roots. Spinal stenosis, disc pain, and z-joint pain are all common in people with this condition.

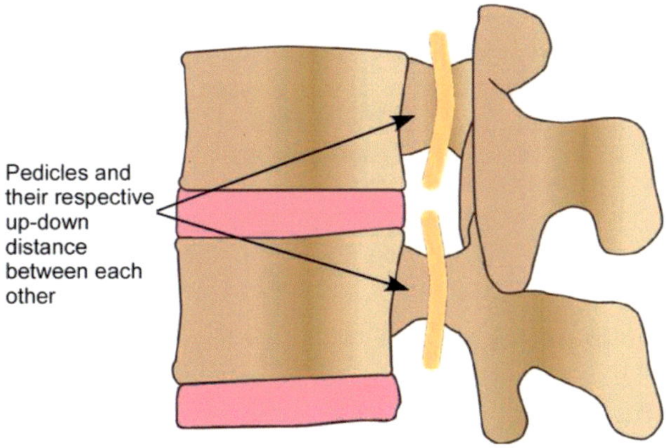

Figure 27: Spinal nerves coursing through central canal and out of invertebral foramen where they are vulnerable to compression and inflammation by the discs up front, decreasing up-down interpedicular distance with disc height shortening, and spurs from the z-joints in the back.

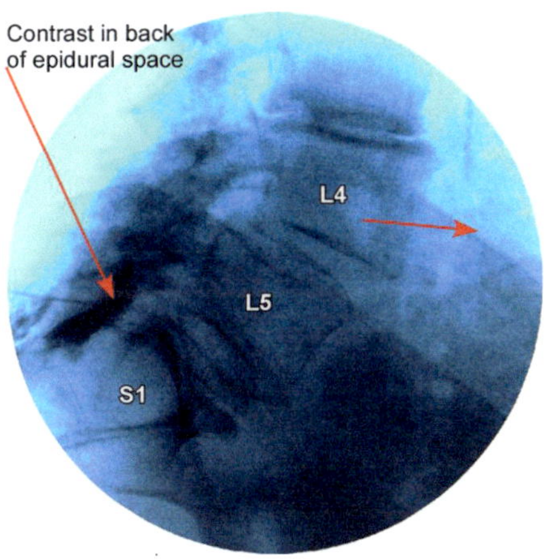

Figure 28: Side view of a lumbar epidural injection in a patient with L4/5 degenerative spondylolisthesis. (L4 is shifted forward in the direction of the red arrow.)

Degenerative spondylolisthesis typically develops after age fifty and is much more common in women—possibly because hormonal changes at menopause cause the spinal ligaments to loosen. People whose lumbar z-joints are angled sharply downward are also at greater risk for developing degenerative spondylolisthesis.

Some people confuse this condition with isthmic lytic spondylolisthesis, a common condition in children that is caused by fractures of the bones surrounding the spinal canal. Both forms of the disease cause forward displacement of the spine. However, unlike the degenerative type, the isthmic lytic form doesn't cause spinal stenosis.

Other Causes

Trauma can cause the vertebral bodies to fracture and fragment into the spinal canal. This is especially common in people with osteoporosis, whose bones may break in response to mild strain during everyday activities. In rare cases, tumors and other abnormal growths can intrude into the spinal canal and cause stenosis.

Recent research suggests a relationship between spinal stenosis and lifestyle-related illness. A Japanese observational study involving five hundred twenty-six patients at sixty-four centers found that hypertension and diabetes were significantly more common in spinal stenosis patients than in the general population. Both illnesses impact blood flow to the spine, which can accelerate the pace of degenerative change. Proper disease management is therefore crucial to ensure the best possible outcomes in people with spinal stenosis.

Does Spinal Stenosis Get Better or Worse Over Time?

Many people, including medical professionals, believe that spinal stenosis is a degenerative disease that causes progressive pain and disability. For this reason, physicians may strongly recommend surgery even when less aggressive treatments are available. However, available evidence does not support this dire view of the condition.

In 2006, researchers published the results of the Michigan Spinal Stenosis Study, which followed thirty-two older patients with MRI-confirmed spinal stenosis for nearly two years. Even though none had surgery, most patients reported significantly less pain and disability as the study progressed. Even more interestingly, the disease showed signs of reversing itself. After twenty months, many participants demonstrated significantly more electrical activity in their paraspinal muscles, and six subjects actually experienced an increase in the diameter of their spinal canals.

The Michigan team noted a number of interesting patterns. For one, patients' initial pain had no impact on their pain twenty months later. Those with severe pain at the beginning of the study were just as likely to improve as those with mild pain. Nor did physiological signs predict outcomes. Patients with narrower spinal canals (as measured on MRI) or less muscle activity (as measured by electrodiagnostic testing) were just as healthy two years later as their counterparts with less severe changes.

Taken together, these findings suggest that people with spinal stenosis tend to improve rather than degenerate over time. This is good news for those who aren't surgical candidates or who wish to explore less invasive treatments before considering surgery.

Diagnosing Spinal Stenosis

In patients with suspected spinal stenosis, diagnostic testing has several goals:

- Confirm that observed stenosis is actually causing symptoms (because in many cases it doesn't).
- Pinpoint other possible contributing pain sources such as z-joint arthritis or disc herniation.
- Distinguish spinal stenosis pain from other types of referred pain (hip joint arthritis, for example, has been shown to cause a similar pattern of referred pain along the L5 spinal nerve distribution).
- Screen for conditions like diabetes and arteriosclerosis that may aggravate spinal stenosis and accelerate degenerative changes. (Good management of these is essential to limit further degeneration and promote favorable outcomes.)
- Uncover tumors, fractures, cauda equina syndrome, and other conditions that require immediate intervention.

Bear in mind that a good diagnosis may take some time—and quite a bit of testing. However, it's important for your doctor to understand the big picture so that you can work together to make good treatment decisions.

Imaging

Imaging modalities like MRI and CT can provide a cross-sectional view of the spinal canal (think of this as looking through the hole of a telescope). When spinal stenosis is present, the canal will appear to be triangular in shape. Narrowing typically appears in the lower, more mobile spine segments (most commonly L4/5 and L5/1).

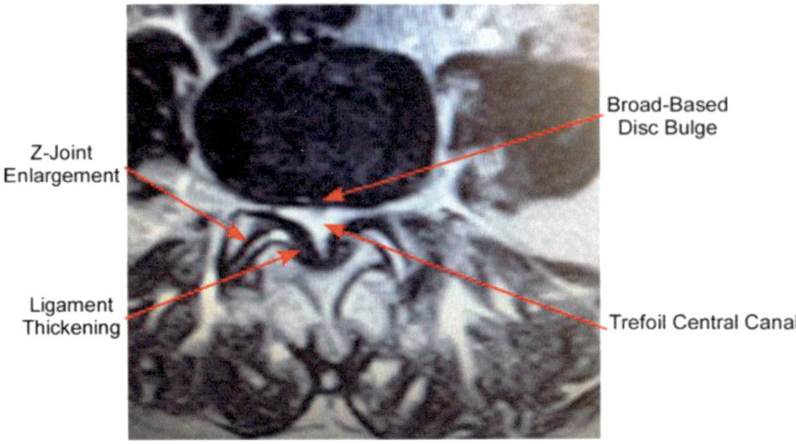

Figure 29: Triangular (trefoil) central canal formed by the above three components in this particular patient.

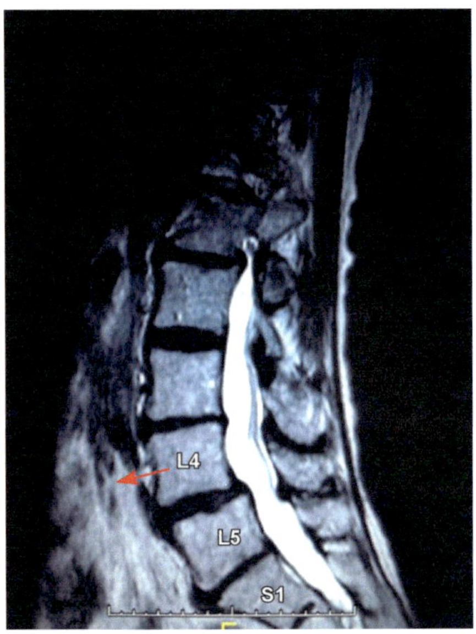

Figure 30: MRI of a seventy-three-year-old man who had difficulty standing and walking due to severe leg pain. The image indicates grade-one spondylolisthesis caused by forward shifting of the L4 vertebral body (in the direction of the red arrow).

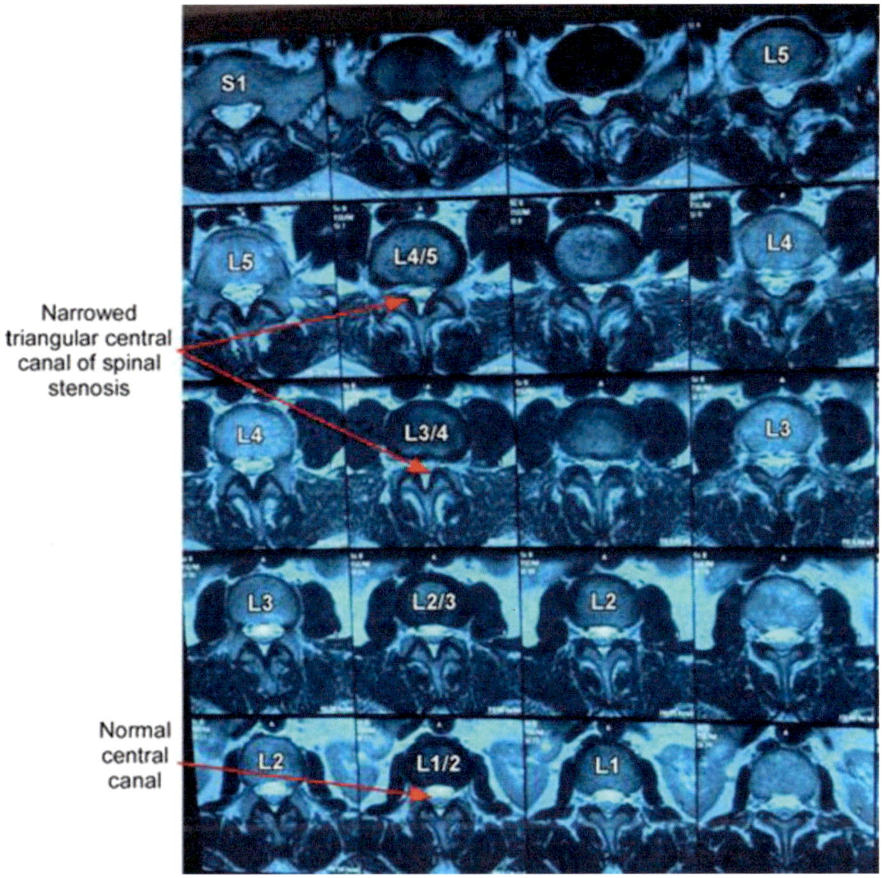

Figure 31: Cross-sectional imaging shows triangular narrowing of the central canal at L4/5 and L3/4 caused by arthritic spurring of the z-joints. Note that the canal is normally sized at L2/3 and L1/2.

To check the degree of spinal stenosis, the radiologist takes measurements of the spinal canal from lateral (side view) images. The descriptor "relative lumbar stenosis" indicates that parts of the spinal canal are less than 12 mm in diameter, while "absolute lumbar stenosis" indicates narrowing to less than 10 mm.

Interestingly, the size of the spinal canal isn't necessarily related to pain or symptoms. Spinal stenosis that is "absolute" in the radiologic sense may cause severe and disabling pain in one person, but no discomfort at all in another. What's more, results of the Michigan Spinal Stenosis Study showed no relationship between MRI findings and the patients' pain and functioning twenty months later. Imaging should therefore be used as a starting point for additional testing and not a definitive diagnostic procedure in itself. In other words, we always treat patients—not pictures.

History and Physical Exam

Spinal stenosis can cause unusual sensations within the affected dermatomes as well as muscle weakness and diminished reflexes in the legs. For more information, see the sections on history and neurological testing in Chapter 7.

Pain due to spinal stenosis may be worsened by standing and walking and relieved by bending slightly forward. Tests such as the crossed straight leg raise are generally not useful in diagnosing spinal stenosis.

Electrodiagnostics

Every time you move, your brain sends an electrical signal through your nervous system to the muscle. These signals are strong and clear when your nerves are functioning well. But if you're experiencing radiculopathy due to compression or irritation of a spinal nerve, they may come through weak or muddled. Ailing nerves may even "misfire" and send signals at the wrong time.

During electrodiagnostic testing, or EDX, your physician uses an external stimulator to test the electrical capacity of the leg nerves. This provides important information about nerve function—both in the peripheral nerves of the lower body and the spinal nerves from which they derive. EDX can measure the size and amplitude of both motor and sensory signals transmitted by your nerves. It can also test the ability of these nerves to carry signals inward toward the spinal cord.

In the most common electrodiagnostic test, your physician places an external stimulator on the skin near the target nerve and delivers a tiny shock. This causes the associated muscle to contract. The time delay between the shock and the muscle response is measured to see how efficiently your nerves are transmitting signals. Results are compared to age norms (and sometimes to speeds on the non-symptomatic side of the body). The shock can cause mild discomfort like burning, tingling, or muscle twitching. However, the test is safe and has no aftereffects.

A related test, **electromyography (EMG)**, records electrical activity within the muscles. The doctor inserts a needle electrode into the target muscle and asks you to contract and relax that muscle. The electrode is wired to a computer that records electrical activity on the screen as a series of peaks and curves. Patterns of weak or unusual electrical activity may signal an underlying nerve problem. By taking readings at several sites, the tester can create an electrical "map" of the muscle group or body part and determine whether the dysfunction originates in a spinal nerve root or further down in a peripheral nerves.

EMG has shown some promise as a diagnostic tool for spinal stenosis. Results of the Michigan Spinal Stenosis Study suggest that mapping of the lumbar paraspinal muscle (which surround the spinal column) was a better predictor of symptomatic stenosis than MRI. However, results had no bearing on future pain or disability.

EMG needle sticks may cause mild pain during the procedure. Afterward, you may notice some fleeting soreness or tingling, which can usually be relieved with over-the-counter painkillers. In some people, the needles cause mild bruising which disappears in a few days.

Treatments for Spinal Stenosis

In the past, most patients with spinal stenosis were referred for surgical evaluation if their symptoms persisted after six months of conservative treatment. However, the growing incidence of spinal stenosis (which primarily affects older people) has prompted research interest in less invasive alternatives, including epidural steroid injections, interspinous process spacers, and minimally invasive decompression. The remainder of this chapter focuses on interventional techniques. For an in-depth discussion of back surgery, see Chapter 9.

Research on several of the treatments below references the Spine Patient Outcomes Research Trial (SPORT), which was conducted in the early 2000s and involved thirteen centers in eleven states. Participants were randomized into surgical and nonsurgical groups. The latter was treated conservatively at their provider's discretion, usually with a combination of epidural steroid injections, physical therapy, counseling, and mild painkillers. SPORT included a lumbar spinal stenosis cohort that is often used as a comparison group when testing the effectiveness of new treatments.

Epidural Steroid Injections

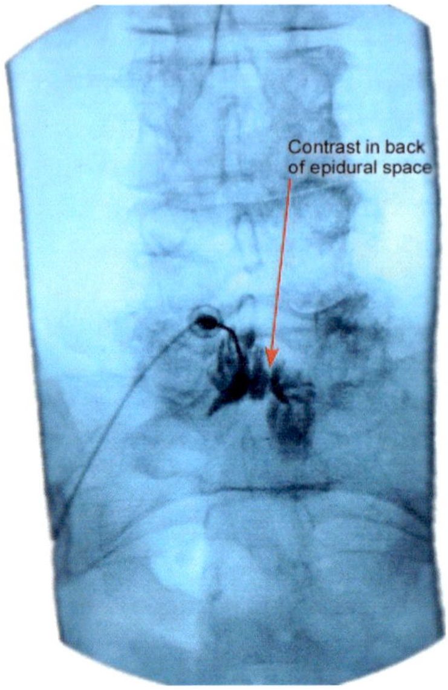

Figure 32: X-ray image (frontal view) and lateral view from Figure 28 of a man who underwent L5/1 interlaminar epidural steroid injection therapy every four months for a year which markedly improved his ability to get around his house.

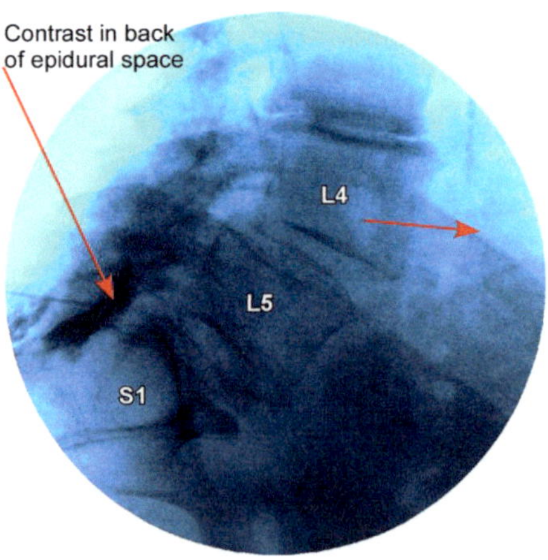

Figure 33: Epidural steroid injections are commonly prescribed for people with spinal stenosis. In a recent survey of spine surgeons, 69 percent of respondents said they consider ESI the next line of treatment after conservative therapy.

In 2012, researchers at Pain Management Center of Paducah (Kentucky) conducted a systematic review of transforaminal epidural steroid injections (the most effective ESI delivery method) as a treatment for low back pain. The authors noted that very few studies existed on the subject, and many of those had significant methodological flaws. They found fair evidence that ESI injections are effective treatments for spinal stenosis pain, and urged further research on the risks and benefits of this approach.

Since the publication of that review, researchers have uncovered even more reason to proceed with caution when considering ESIs. A 2013 study published in Spine compared outcomes for sixty lumbar spinal stenosis patients who received ESI during the first three months of the SPORT study with two hundred seven who did not. Over time, the ESI group fared worse, experiencing significantly more pain and disability across four years of follow-up. Furthermore, ESI patients who later elected to have back surgery had longer operation times and hospital stays. Researchers hypothesized that the steroid and anesthetic injections may actually aggravate spinal stenosis, though they note that further research is needed to confirm this.

Given the evidence, patients and their physicians should carefully discuss the potential risks and benefits when considering ESI as a treatment for spinal stenosis. For a more detailed description of the procedure itself, see Chapter 4.

Lumbar Interspinous Process Spacers (IPSs)

These devices are placed between the spinous processes of adjacent vertebrae to hold the spine in a stable, slightly flexed position. For people with spinal stenosis, this mimics the pain-relieving effects of bending forward while allowing the patient to stand and sit normally. Examples of IPSs include X-STOP, Coflex, the Wallis implant, and DIAM. Implantation requires very simple surgery that can be performed under local anesthetic.

Do IPSs work?

An early systematic review carried out in the United Kingdom found that IPSs have beneficial effects on spine mechanics, and that preliminary trials generally demonstrate advantages over conservative therapy. However, given the growing popularity of these devices (which are being marketed for a number of uses not supported by research), the team urged additional controlled, randomized trials to guide clinical decision-making.

The best-studied IPS is the Medtronic **X-STOP**, which is FDA approved for the treatment of spinal stenosis pain in patients fifty and older who are experiencing neurogenic claudication. In FDA approval trials, 45 percent of patients treated with X-STOP demonstrated an overall improvement in symptom severity, 44 percent showed better physical function, and 73 percent said they were satisfied or very satisfied with the results. However, this study was widely criticized for including data from an institution affiliated with the device manufacturer. Results of later trials have shown more modest benefits.

A 2011 study published in Spine examined X-STOP's cost-effectiveness compared with conservative care and laminectomy surgery. Participants who received the X-STOP implant as a treatment for moderate spinal stenosis pain were followed for two years. Researchers concluded that when compared with conservative treatment, X-STOP provided better long-term quality of life that justified its somewhat higher cost. When compared to laminectomy surgery, X-STOP was both less expensive and provided better long-term quality of life. This is good news for patients who are reluctant to have surgery and are looking for less invasive treatments.

Critics of IPSs have raised concerns about the possibility of fractures. The spinous processes are relatively delicate bones that are not designed to sustain compressional loading—especially in older people who tend to have lower bone mass. Though very few fractures were noted in initial safety trials, these relied on plain x-rays. In a later study, more powerful CT scans revealed fractures in eleven of thirty-eight patients treated with IPSs. While not always painful, fractures were associated with less relief and poorer patient satisfaction one year later. Larger studies are needed to explore the problem further.

Is an IPS right for you?

You might benefit from an IPS surgery if you have confirmed spinal stenosis at one or two spinal levels and leg pain relieved by forward flexion. Results are generally best in people with mild to moderate impairment who can still perform some of their daily activities. Because spinal stenosis pain tends to improve over time, you should undergo six months of conservative treatment before considering an IPS. Finally, IPS is not safe for people with severe osteoporosis, past spine surgery, or conditions like spondylolisthesis (which could cause spine instability).

Risks and side effects.

IPS implants are generally safe. In their FDA approval application, X-STOP's manufacturers reported adverse effects in about 3 percent of cases. The most common problems involved the device dislodging or moving, which required additional surgery to correct. Recent concerns have been raised about the high rate of fractures in ISPs recipients.

What to expect

IPS surgery is usually performed on an outpatient basis, meaning you can go home the same day. Your doctor will use local or general anesthetic, depending on the type of device, your health, and your personal preferences. During the procedure, the surgeon makes a two-to-three-inch incision above the spinal level to be treated, moves the device into position under x-ray guidance, and attaches it to the surrounding bones.

Aftercare

In most cases, your health care provider will encourage you to get up and walk as soon as you can after surgery. Some soreness at the site is normal but can usually be managed with over-the-counter pain medications. You'll need to follow some activity restrictions for two to six weeks after surgery, which may prohibit stair climbing, lifting, and certain sports. Your doctor may also recommend light exercise or physical therapy to help restore your mobility and strength.

Minimally Invasive Lumbar Decompression (mild)

For many years, surgical decompression, or laminectomy, was the only way to permanently relieve nerve compression due to spinal stenosis. However, surgery is associated with high complication rates and long recovery times, especially in older patients. Advances like endoscopes and microscopes have made the process a bit easier, but it remains a major operation requiring an overnight hospital stay.

Fortunately, a minimally invasive treatment called mild (minimally invasive lumbar decompression) is producing excellent results for some patients while allowing them to avoid the risks of surgery. During mild, the surgeon uses a kit of sterile, single-use tools to remove tiny pieces of ligament and bone from the constricted spinal canal. Mild requires only a tiny incision, takes less than an hour, and is performed on an outpatient basis under light sedation. Patients almost always go home the same day.

Does mild work?

Repeated studies have shown mild to be safe and effective in treating patients with mild to moderate spinal stenosis pain. A multi-year study of fifty-eight patients treated with mild at the Cleveland Clinic found no complications from the procedure. (By contrast, up to 25 percent of laminectomy surgeries involve complications like dural punctures, bleeding into the epidural space, or infection.) A systematic safety review of three hundred seventy-three patients found that 80 percent experienced significant improvement in their symptoms, and 74 percent were satisfied or very satisfied with the results after one year. These outcomes were comparable to those observed in open surgery patients during the SPORT trial.

Is mild right for me?

Mild may be an option for you if:

- You have spinal stenosis pain confirmed by diagnostic imaging.
- Your condition is mainly caused by thickening of the ligaments.
- Your symptoms do not resolve after six months of conservative therapy.

Risks and side effects

Mild has an excellent safety record, and complications are rare. However, it doesn't work for everyone. A minority of patients continues to have leg pain. The current efficacy studies thus far, however, are inconclusive.

What to Expect

During mild, you're given a light sedative and your spine area is numbed with a local anesthetic. Next, your doctor injects contrast agent into the epidural space to help visualize the tools under x-ray guidance. Working through a tiny incision just a few millimeters long, the doctor gently compresses the nerves to one side of the spinal canal to create a safe working area. He or she then uses the tiny mild tools to remove tiny bits of bone and ligament tissue. Afterward, the incision is closed with a Steri-Strip. No stitches are needed, and the whole procedure takes less than an hour.

Aftercare

After mild, you may have some back pain, which can usually be managed with over-the-counter medications like Tylenol.

Benita: Weighing the Options

By the time Benita was diagnosed with spinal stenosis, she'd suffered through six years of intense, unrelenting pain and ineffective treatment. Although she appeared to be a surgical candidate, she was physically weak from lack of activity and suffering from serious depression. We therefore decided to take a less aggressive approach for the time being.

Because epidural steroid injections had helped Benita in the past, we decided to give them another try. After the first treatment, she was able to walk around her apartment, and even stood up long enough to cook dinner. Within two weeks, she'd enrolled in an aquatic therapy program, which helped to gently rehabilitate her weakened muscles and joints.

For the next three years, Benita continued the periodic steroid injections with good results. She regained her ability to sit and walk for short periods and was no longer dependent on an aide at home. She enjoyed her sessions in the pool and befriended several of the women she met there. As her quality of life improved, her depression gradually lifted. She felt alive for the first time in years.

After three years of steroid injections, Benita seemed strong enough to take the next step toward recovery, and I referred her to an excellent spine surgeon in our area for a preliminary consultation.

Key Points

- Spinal stenosis is the most common spine condition diagnosed in older adults.
- Degenerative changes to the intervertebral discs, z-joints, and spinal ligaments (the latter of which thicken with age) often cause the spinal canal to shift and narrow. This can compress the nearby spinal nerves, resulting in significant leg pain.
- In the past, most patients were referred for surgery if symptoms persisted after six months of conservative therapy. However, new minimally invasive treatments such as interspinous process spacers and mild offer alternatives for some.

Many patients with spinal stenosis do go on to have back surgery, which is discussed in detail in the next chapter.

9

LOW BACK SURGERY: RISKS AND REWARDS

Benita (whose story began in Chapter 8) was open to the idea of surgery. After nearly a decade of chronic, disabling pain, it seemed like her best hope for a normal life. Though her spinal stenosis pain had responded somewhat to epidural steroid injections and aquatic therapy, she still had trouble sitting and walking for more than fifteen minutes or so. At my recommendation, she visited a spine surgeon to explore more aggressive treatments.

After examining Benita, the surgeon told her that she was a good candidate for a laminectomy, an operation that removes part of the "roof" of the spinal canal. If all went well, she would be free of leg pain and able to sit and walk for as long as she liked. Of course, there were also drawbacks. Because of her age, she'd be at greater risk for complications, and full recovery was likely to take several months. She'd also need to commit to intensive rehabilitation and physical therapy during this period.

Benita was hesitant. Despite her recent gains, she wasn't satisfied with her current lifestyle. She wanted to drive her car, work in her garden, and travel with her husband. On the other hand, she knew enough people who'd undergone back surgery to realize what she might be in for. She'd been through so much already. Was an operation really worth the pain and hassle?

Back Surgery: What's Involved?

Back surgery has always been controversial. In its early years, high rates of failure and complications made it a treatment of last resort. "No operation in any field of surgery leaves in its wake more human wreckage than surgery on the lumbar disc," wrote pioneering orthopedic surgeons Anthony F. DePalma and Richard H. Rothman in 1969.

Fortunately, we've come a long way in four decades. New techniques have made back surgery safer and more effective than ever. We also have a far better understanding of which patients are likely to benefit from surgery—and which might do just as well with more conservative care.

Thus far, this book has focused on conservative and minimally invasive treatments for low back pain. I've saved surgical procedures for last because they're usually reserved for patients whose pain hasn't responded to less aggressive interventions. Although it's still used as a last resort, surgery can be very effective when prescribed appropriately and according to evidence-based guidelines. I've had patients who resisted the idea of surgery, but were ultimately so pleased by the results they wished they'd had it sooner.

Back surgery is most likely to be successful when:

- You're in relatively good physical and mental health.
- Less aggressive treatments haven't helped (or aren't available).
- You've undergone a rigorous diagnostic process to pinpoint the source of your pain and rule out other painful conditions.
- A skilled, experienced surgeon is available to perform the procedure.
- Research suggests that your type of back pain responds better to surgical treatment than to conservative therapy.

Let's start by taking a look at the most common forms of back surgery: discectomy, laminectomy, spinal fusion, and total disc replacement. Later in the chapter, we'll discuss how back surgery stacks up against conservative care as a treatment for low back pain.

Discectomy

As we've discussed previously, a herniated disc can compress the nerve root, causing both mechanical and nerve pain. Discectomy relieves this pressure by removing bulging or extruded disc material from the epidural space.

Discectomy performed under microscopic guidance provides the surgeon with an enhanced view of the disc and surrounding structures. Advances such as endoscopes (tiny, lighted tubes with attached cameras) allow surgery to be performed through smaller incisions, which usually means less pain and faster healing afterward. The exact technique depends on the location and type of your disc herniation as well as your surgeon's training and preferences.

Does discectomy work?

Discectomy has been shown to provide significant pain relief in a majority of patients with leg pain due to disc herniation. A Japanese study published in 2001 reviewed the records of 72 patients with confirmed disc herniation who'd undergone discectomy ten or more years ago. About 70 percent experienced significant pain reduction lasting at least a decade. In most cases, surgeons were able to preserve the height of the herniated disc, which was associated with better long-term outcomes.

Recent technological advances may enhance the benefits of discectomy. A 2006 study conducted in China showed excellent outcomes for eight hundred seventy-three disc herniation patients treated with **endoscopic discectomy**. During surgery, these patients experienced only a third of the blood loss demonstrated by the control group, which underwent standard open discectomy. The endoscopic group also had shorter hospital stays and quicker recovery times. Both open and endoscopic patients experienced similar rates of surgical complications (4 to 5 percent), including spinal cord injuries, disc infections, and wound infections. At thirty months follow up, about 90 percent of patients in both groups demonstrated good or excellent outcomes.

Traditionally, a surgeon performing discectomy accesses the damaged disc from the rear or side of the spine. However, scar tissue sometimes blocks this approach in patients who have undergone previous back surgeries. A relatively new technique called **endoscopic transforaminal discectomy (ETD)** allows the surgeon to bypass the scarred area and access the diseased disc endoscopically through the foramen. Hoogland and colleagues found an 86 percent satisfaction rating among recurrent disc herniation patients treated with ETD. At two years follow-up, these patients reported significant pain relief and gains in functional ability, and about a third felt fully recovered. Complication rates were found to be similar to other types of discectomy.

Risks and side effects

The success of discectomy appears to depend somewhat on the surgeon's skill and experience. This is especially true when advances like endoscopes are used. Operating under endoscopic guidance is very different than working with an optical microscope and requires extensive training. The authors of the Chinese study on endoscopic discectomy reported that the incidence of complications fell markedly during the study period—presumably because the skill of the surgeon and surgical assistant increased in the course of performing over eight hundred identical surgeries. (This is one reason it's a good idea to seek out the most experienced specialist you can find when considering back surgery.)

Some long-term studies of discectomy have noted high rates of lingering back pain years down the road. The Japanese study cited above found mild to moderate residual back pain in about 75 percent of discectomy patients. In most cases, this did not keep subjects from their daily activities. However, about 13 percent of participants experienced severe residual pain. This was most common in younger patients (under thirty-five) with evidence of advanced disc degeneration at the time of surgery. The team theorized that this finding might be related to the participants' activities before and after surgery (team sports or heavy lifting at work, for example).

Finally, disc herniation recurs after surgery in about 10 to 15 percent of people treated with discectomy. About 12.5 percent of the subjects in the Japanese study had repeat herniation within ten years. Interestingly, recurrence was most common in the group with the best initial outcomes (i.e., preserved disc height and significant pain relief). Hoogland and colleagues' ETD trial found a recurrence rate of 4.6 percent over two years.

What to expect

In most cases, discectomy is performed under general anesthesia. Your surgeon makes a small incision (about two to three centimeters long) in the back and gently retracts the spinal muscles to one side. Small bits of bone and ligament may be removed to expose the disc. Protruding disc parts are "trimmed" and fragments of disc material removed from the disc itself and epidural space. The entire procedure takes about an hour. The surgery may be performed as an outpatient, although most people spend at least one night in the hospital after discectomy. Your doctor will prescribe pain medication to take as needed after the procedure.

Aftercare

Though you will have some activity restrictions for a few weeks, gentle exercise like walking will promote healing. Some people also benefit from physical therapy during the recovery period.

Spinal Fusion Surgery (Arthrodesis), Laminectomy Surgery

Some operations result in structural weakness within the spine. In cases of advanced disc degeneration or disc herniation, the surgeon may actually remove most of the diseased disc. People with spinal stenosis may undergo laminotomy, in which bits of bone and ligament are removed to create more room inside the spinal canal, or laminectomy, in which the entire roof of the spinal canal at a particular segment is removed. In these cases, the surgeon may choose to "fuse" two or more vertebra together to prevent instability that could injure the spinal cord. In some cases, fusion is also used to prevent motion that could compress or irritate the nerve roots.

To achieve fusion, the surgeon grafts the ends of the surrounding vertebrae together, often with donor bone or material harvested from the patient's own hipbone. Screws and rods are attached to provide extra support and prevent motion.

Does spinal fusion work?

In recent years, the number of spinal fusion surgeries performed in the United States has increased dramatically. However, the procedure remains controversial. A 2009 systematic review by the American Pain Society found little evidence that spinal fusion is any better than conservative care as a treatment for low back pain caused by a painful disc.

Does that mean spinal fusion should never be used in such cases? Not necessarily. As you'll recall from Chapter 4, discogenic pain is difficult to diagnose. Disc pain is often assumed to be the problem when in fact the true pain generator lies elsewhere. Hence, failure to adhere to strict patient selection procedures could explain the high rate of surgical "failures" in existing studies.

Two years after the American Pain Society's review, a Japanese team achieved more promising results in a group of forty-one patients with discogenic low back pain. In this case, patients were only considered for spinal fusion if their disc pain was confirmed by disc stimulation ie provocative lumbar discography. After two years, the group treated with spinal fusion surgery was experiencing significantly better outcomes than the control group treated with conservative care. Researchers concluded that fusion surgery can indeed benefit carefully selected patients with discogenic low back pain.

In people with symptomatic spinal stenosis, the American Pain Society study found that fusion surgery was moderately superior to nonsurgical treatment, and that benefits were apparent up to two years later.

What are the risks of spinal fusion?

Potential complications of spinal fusion surgery include infection, poor healing, and lingering pain at the "harvest" site (if the patient's own bone is removed for grafting), bleeding, neuralgia issues including weakness or numbness, spinal fluid leak, recurrence of disc Herniation, resistant or worsening symptoms, medical issues including deep venous thrombosis (blood clot in legs) with association pulmonary embolism (blood clot to the lungs), myocardial infarction, stroke or even death.

Fusion changes the way the spine moves and bears force. Over time, this can cause adjacent segment degeneration (ASD), a condition in which these mechanical changes accelerate wear and tear along the edges of the fused area. ASD leads to increased rates of z-joint arthritis and internal disc disruption syndrome and can cause significant pain and disability down the road.

A systematic review conducted by Chinese researchers evaluated the prevalence of ASD in patients who underwent neck and low back surgery, including lumbar fusion and total disc replacement. Their exhaustive study included the results of ninety-four published papers involving over thirty-four thousand participants worldwide. Results suggested that 27 percent of lumbar spine surgery patients eventually showed signs of ASD, and about 8.5 percent experienced pain due to the condition. These findings strongly suggest that the risk of ASD be weighed when considering lumbar spine fusion.

What to expect

Spinal fusion is performed under general anesthesia. Depending on the location to be fused, your surgeon will make an incision in your back, side, or abdomen. An additional incision sometimes is made if bone will be harvested from your hipbone or pelvis.

Where appropriate, biologic agents including bone morphogenic proteins (BMPs) may be used to stimulate grafting of your vertebrae. BMPs are grown in a lab using recombinant DNA technology. They eliminate the need to harvest bone from other parts of your body and have been shown to be very effective in fusion procedures although recent studies have shown several possible complications associated with their use including excess bone formation, radiculopathy or even cancer. Other biologic agents may be used to supplement bone harvest and diminish the risks of theses potential problems.

Once the vertebrae are grafted together, screws, plates, and other mechanical devices are added to strengthen the fused segment.

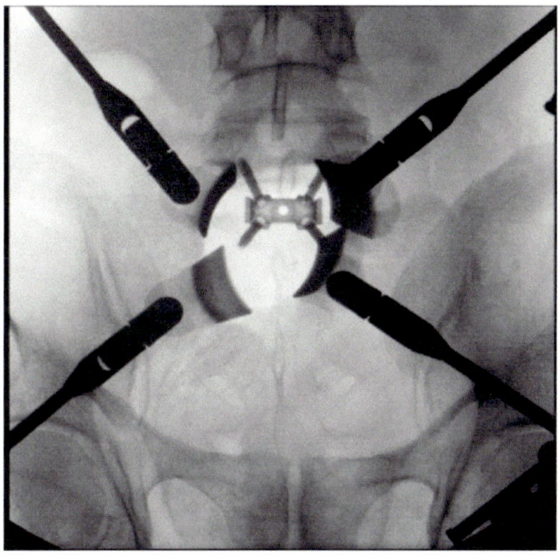

Figure 34: Anterior lumbar interbody fusion (ALIF) allows the disc space left after the disc is removed to be fused by approaching the spine from the front (i.e., via the abdomen) rather than placing the fusion device through the back or posterior part of the spine (as done in a posterior interbody fusion). This surgery is typically performed along with a vascular surgeon who moves the blood vessel out of the way to allow disc access for implantation of the fusion prosthesis on the left.

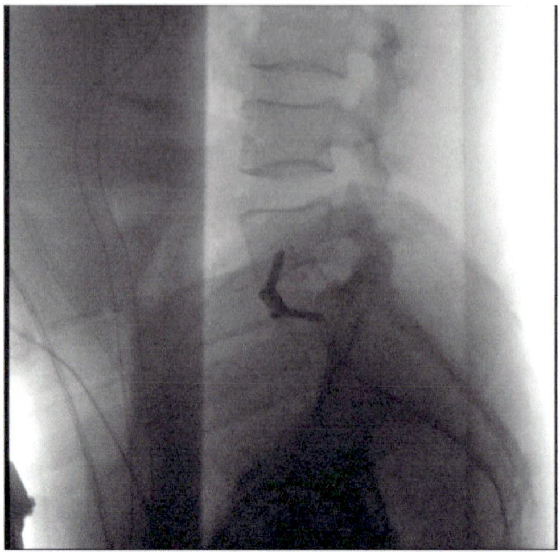

Figure 35: Lateral (side) view of a fusion device placed through the front of the spine, on the right

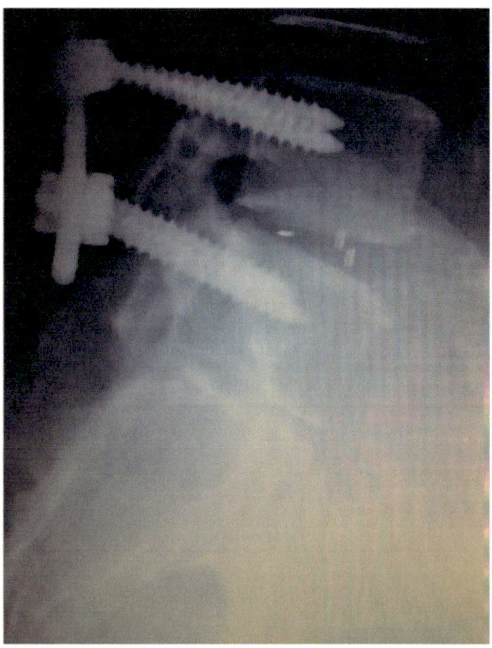

Figure 36:

Posterior Lumbar Interbody Fusion Surgery Description

After the muscles are peeled off of the lamina (the roof of the spinal column), the lamina itself is taken off to allow access to the disc. The disc is then removed from the disc space, and one of many different types of prostheses is placed in the space. Note the pedicle screws being placed through the pedicles into the vertebral bodies. Fusion is generally performed to stop the motion of a painful disc or to stabilize the spine in the case of a fracture, infection, or tumor

Aftercare

After spinal fusion, you can expect to spend a couple of days in the hospital. Pain at the incision site is common and can usually be controlled with medications. You will need to follow activity restrictions and possibly wear a brace for several weeks while your spine heals. Physical therapy is often prescribed to help you regain your range of motion and adjust your posture after fusion.

Total Disc Replacement (Disc Arthroplasty)

Total disc replacement may offer an alternative to spinal fusion that preserves normal spine motion and minimizes ASD down the road. After removing the problematic disc, the surgeon inserts a prosthesis between the vertebral bodies. In theory, this restores disc height, which can help relieve nerve root compression caused by sinking of the foramina i.e. the holes where the nerves exit the spine. Examples of available disc replacement devices include Prodisc II, CHARITE III, Maverick, and Flexicore.

Does disc replacement work?

Total disc replacement appears to be safe and effective in certain patients—at least in the short term. A study conducted in Australia followed 122 patients treated with the CHARITE artificial disc for a minimum of two years. All patients were diagnosed with single-level discogenic pain, which was confirmed through history, physical examination, imaging, disc stimulation and (where indicated) electrodiagnostic testing. To be considered for the study, patients first had to complete at least twelve months of conservative care with emphasis on physical therapy.

This carefully selected group demonstrated significant improvements in back pain, leg pain, and overall function from three months onward. At all times, at least 85 percent of patients rated their satisfaction level with the procedure as "good" or "excellent." While the authors did not report on longer-term complications like ASD, they noted that the procedure appeared to preserve motion at the operative segment.

While these results are promising, much more research is needed before total disc replacement can be recommended without reservations. A 2012 Cochrane Review compared the effectiveness of disc replacement to that of spinal fusion surgery for the treatment of discogenic back pain. Researchers identified seven randomized controlled trials, all of which they deemed methodologically flawed. Several involved potential conflicts of interest because they were partially funded by device manufacturers or other interested parties. Hence, all of the review's conclusions were based on lower-quality evidence.

The Cochrane reviewers found that compared with fusion surgery, disc replacement showed statistically significant reductions in pain and disability. However, these findings weren't clinically relevant—in other words, the improvements, while genuine, were probably too small to be meaningful to patients. They also noted that none of the studies adequately addressed ASD or other long-term complications. The team therefore urged physicians to use caution when recommending total disc replacement, stating that more research is needed to explore its long-term effects.

Risks and side effects

Disc replacement is not safe for people who have:

- Spinal instability (including degenerative spondylolisthesis)
- Severe z-joint arthritis
- Osteoporosis
- Previous fusion at the target level

Some trials of total disc replacement have raised concerns about long-term complications. One, a Norwegian study published in 2012 by Hellum and colleagues, compared the course of spinal degeneration in fifty-nine patients who underwent disc replacement surgery and fifty-seven treated with physical therapy. After two years, the surgical group showed no evidence of ASD. However, they did have significantly more z-joint arthritis at the implant level than the control group (34 percent versus 4 percent respectively). Like the Cochrane team, the authors concluded that further research is needed to explore the long-term effects of total disc replacement surgery.

What to expect

Disc replacement is performed under general anesthetic. Working under x-ray guidance, the surgeon makes a small incision in the abdomen, removes the degraded part of the disc, and inserts the prosthetic. In most cases normal loading of the spine holds the prosthetic in place, so there is no need for screws or plates. Surgery usually takes one to three hours.

As with other back surgeries, total disc replacement requires an overnight hospital stay. Afterwards you will need to follow activity restrictions and may benefit from physical therapy as your back heals.

Is Surgery Really Better than Other Treatments?

Surgery has an impressive track record when it comes to treating some types of back pain. For others, more conservative treatments may be a wiser course. Surgery is generally considered only if conservative treatments fail.

For Discogenic Pain Due to Degenerative Changes

The American Pain Society study found that spinal fusion may have some benefits over standard conservative care but was less effective then intensive rehabilitation and behavior modification. For further discussion, see the spinal fusion section above.

For Disc Herniation

The American Pain Society study found good evidence that standard open discectomy and microdiscectomy are superior to nonoperative treatment, at least in the short term. There was not enough evidence available to compare total disc replacement to conservative care. Researchers noted that disc herniation patients tended to improve with or without surgery, and that the short-term advantages of surgery faded with time.

These findings support those of an earlier study by Osterman and colleagues, which compared the effectiveness of microdiscectomy and conservative treatment in fifty people with leg pain due to disc herniation.

During the early weeks of the trial, the surgical group saw more improvements. However, two years later, no significant differences remained between the surgical and control groups in regards to pain intensity, disability, and quality of life.

Osterman's and the APS's findings are somewhat contradicted by those of the SPORT study. An analysis of 1,191 patients with confirmed disc herniation found that those who underwent surgery experienced less leg and low-back pain at follow up. What's more, the surgical group was more likely to report significant pain relief or no pain at all throughout the follow-up period. Though the relative benefits of surgery lessened over time, they were still statistically significant two years later. Researchers concluded that while both approaches reduce pain, "Surgery is more likely to lead to greater or complete relief."

An analysis by Tosteson and colleagues examined the cost-effectiveness of surgical versus non-operative care among patients in SPORT's disc herniation cohort. The study included seven hundred seventy-five patients who underwent open discectomy and four hundred sixteen treated conservatively at a physician's discretion. They found that surgery was moderately cost-effective at two years follow-up, suggesting that its medical and quality-of-life benefits outweighed its greater initial cost.

For Symptomatic Spinal Stenosis

As noted above, the American Pain Society study found good evidence that laminectomy with or without fusion achieved better outcomes than non-operative therapy for up to two years. The relative benefits of surgery diminished over time (though less dramatically than in people with disc herniation).

Benita: Conquering the Great Wall

Two years ago, Benita underwent laminectomy surgery. Due to complications, she spent a week in the hospital and took several months to recover. However, she was mentally prepared for these setbacks and very motivated to improve. She attended physical therapy and diligently followed her at-home exercise program. Though the full benefits of surgery took several months to realize, she and Raul celebrated every small milestone.

Today Benita can stand and walk as long as she likes and is enjoying an active retirement. Her garden is once again the envy of the block. When zucchini is in season, she rides her bicycle from house to house to deliver the surplus harvest to her neighbors. She also serves as a spiritual care volunteer at the hospital where she used to work. "All those years of pain have definitely given me perspective on what the patients are going through," she says.

Last year, at the age of seventy, Benita traveled to Beijing with Raul to visit the Great Wall of China. It was a dream they had all but given up on. "Two years ago, I couldn’t even sit up on the couch, much less on an airplane for fourteen hours," she says. "Now, thanks to my surgery, I walked all over that wall. I even skipped the cable car and climbed the stairs to the top."

The Bottom Line

Having back surgery is a big decision that warrants a careful conversation with the best surgeon you can find. There’s no magic formula for determining whether surgery is the best option for you. When discussing the possibility, you and your surgeon should consider:

- **Likelihood of improvement without surgery.** Studies show that people with disc herniation (and to a lesser degree spinal stenosis) tend to improve over time, even without surgery.

- **The cause of your back pain.** Surgery is more effective at treating some types of back pain (disc herniation, for example) than others.

- **Diagnostic confidence.** Surgery is more likely to be successful when the source of the pain has been confirmed by thorough testing.

- **Practical considerations.** You must be prepared to deal with costs, activity restrictions, and the need for physical therapy after surgery.

- **Your physical and mental health.** Some chronic conditions can increase the risk of complications during surgery. Severe depression is associated with poorer surgical outcomes.

- **Short-term risks.** All surgeries carry the risk of rare but potentially serious complications.

- **Long-term risks.** Lumbar spine surgery carries a risk of long-term complications like ASD.

- **Available alternatives.** Do you have access to less aggressive treatments that are likely to provide the same benefits as surgery?

For certain patients, there's no doubt that back surgery can be a lifesaver. But what if it doesn't work? In the next chapter, we'll discuss your options if back surgery fails to provide the relief you need.

10

FAILED BACK SURGERY SYNDROME: WHAT NOW?

John, thirty-one, a high school teacher and football coach, was the guy his friends always called when they needed a hand. Though he'd been an elite athlete in college and had played a season with a professional football team, he remained extremely humble and down-to-earth. He always made helping others a priority, whether he was driving his beloved grandmother to the doctor, moving a friend, or babysitting his three nephews.

In the spring of 2010, John was cleaning his mom's gutters when he slipped on some loose leaves and tumbled off the roof. He downplayed his accident at first, saying he was lucky to have gotten away with nothing more serious than bruises. But within a week, he saw his family doctor complaining of severe pain in his lower back. An MRI revealed several herniated discs.

When six months of physical therapy failed to relieve John's pain, he was referred to a surgeon and eventually underwent a two-level lumbar fusion. After the operation, he waited anxiously for normality to return. Instead, he got worse. Every step set off deep, throbbing back pain that eventually spread to his legs. He could barely climb the stairs to his walk-up apartment. Though he hated the idea of taking narcotic medications, it was the only way he could stand long enough to coach his players through a practice.

The decision to have surgery had not been easy for John, He felt that by taking time off, he'd let his students and players down. When the operation failed, he was uncharacteristically angry with everyone—his doctors, family members, friends—who had assured him that surgery would fix everything. He wished he'd listened to his gut and done more research instead of rushing into the procedure.

When John came to me for a second opinion, he brought along previous imaging studies, which showed a high level of spinal degeneration. This isn't unusual in younger people who have played contact sports. As I listened to him talk, however, I realized just how perfunctory his diagnosis had been. His pain could have come from any number of problems that showed up on MRI—or none of them. No one had referred him for disc stimulation before surgery, which would have confirmed with confidence whether any of his disc bulges were actually painful.

When I explained all of this to John, he was justifiably angry. Once he understood that many physicians still hold misconceptions about imaging and disc stimulation, he felt better and was able to focus on next steps.

Unfortunately, as is sometimes the case with a spine like John's, a clear-cut diagnosis moving forward proved to be elusive. Steroid injections, nerve blocks, and disc stimulation yielded inconsistent results. No test pointed to a clear pain generator that could be treated with revision surgery. However, a new MRI did show a mass of scar tissue forming around the nerves near the fusion site.

By this point, John had been through a lot and was beginning to feel hopeless. I reassured him that even though the surgery itself had produced disappointing results, he still had options. His post-surgery pain was an obstacle, not a dead end.

Failed Back Surgery Syndrome: What Is It?

Failed back surgery syndrome, or FBSS, is chronic back and leg pain that develops or persists after back surgery. It can happen after any kind of operation, though it's most often associated with laminectomy (and sometimes called postlaminectomy syndrome).

FBSS pain may be apparent immediately after surgery or may appear after the patient has been symptom-free for months or years. Depending on the mechanism involved, it may be dull, achy, or sharp, and may appear in the back, legs, or buttocks. If nerve roots are compressed or irritated, the person may experience sensory abnormalities, muscle weakness and diminished reflexes.

How Common Is FBSS?

Some ongoing pain is pretty common after back surgery and doesn't necessarily mean the operation has failed. A retrospective Japanese study that followed up with patients ten or more years after discectomy found that that about 62 percent had mild to moderate residual low back pain. An additional 13 percent reported severe pain. This was most common in people under thirty-five who (like John) showed extensive spinal degeneration prior to surgery.

What Causes FBSS?

After an operation, tough scar tissue often forms at the surgical site. In some cases, this fibrous mass can compress the spinal nerve roots and take up space in the spinal canal. Scarring can also block the normal incision routes, making repeat surgeries more difficult.

Certain patients are at increased risk of developing FBSS. Some medical conditions (notably diabetes, vascular diseases, and autoimmune diseases) interfere with the healing process and promote the formation of scar tissue. People who smoke cigarettes are also more prone to FBSS, possibly due to their reduced bone metabolism and circulation.

Fortunately, technological advances like minimally invasive surgery and endoscopes are making operations less traumatic, which decreases the likelihood of scarring. For example, endoscopic transforaminal discectomy (ETD) allows your surgeon to access your discs via the spinal foramen (as opposed to through the back side of the spine, as happens in open discectomy). This dramatically reduces post-surgical scarring, decreasing the likelihood of FBSS and making future surgeries safer and easier.

Where to Go From Here?

FBSS can be an enormous letdown after the risks and hassles of back surgery. However, like other types of back pain, it's usually treatable. Mild cases can often be managed with conservative care. When pain is severe or disabling, spinal cord stimulation may be used to correct the problem.

Spinal Cord Stimulation

A spinal cord stimulator (SCS) is a device that uses tiny pulses of electricity to disrupt the transmission of pain signals through the spinal cord to the brain. It consists of stimulating electrodes, which are implanted in the epidural space and wired to a generator beneath the skin of the abdomen or buttocks.

Leg pain due to FBSS is the most common reason people undergo spinal cord stimulation in the United States. The device is also used as a first-line treatment for radicular pain, especially in people who are poor surgical candidates. Other chronic pain conditions, such as angina, peripheral vascular disease or peripheral neuropathy may also respond to SCS.

How does SCS work?

The exact mechanism of action behind SCS remains a mystery. Certain kinds of sensory stimuli seem to shut off columns within the back side of the spinal cord that transmit pain. More recent studies indicate that SCS may stimulate the spinal cord to release GABA, serotonin, and adenosine—chemicals that help to soothe nerve pain.

Is SCS effective?

SCS provides significant and lasting relief in up to 60 percent of patients with chronic pain, according to the website of the American Association of Neurological Surgeons. When used to treat FBSS, it's most effective if:

- The failed surgery was recent (within the past three years)
- The main complaint is burning nerve pain that radiates into the extremities
- The patient is free of psychological problems (especially depression)

While SCS is best studied as a treatment for radicular pain, recent technological advances may allow people with simple, non-radiating low back pain to benefit as well (though benefits are not as clear-cut for this group).

So, when it comes to lasting relief, how does SCS stack up against surgery? Unfortunately, we don't have much high-quality evidence on the subject—probably due to the difficulty of designing a suitable experiment. However, at least one randomized, controlled study has compared outcomes of twenty-four FBSS patients treated with spinal cord stimulation to twenty-six who had additional surgery. SCS achieved significant pain relief (greater than 50 percent) in 38 percent of patients. Only 12 percent who had a second operation showed comparable improvement.

While more controlled trials of SCS are needed, many physicians have published case studies on the subject, creating a sizable body of evidence that covers thousands of patients (including some who were followed for ten years or longer). Based on their analysis of these reports, the authors of a 2004 systematic review found no evidence of major adverse effects due to SCS, suggesting a good safety record for the procedure.

Is SCS right for you?

Before considering SCS, you should complete at least six months of conservative therapy, which may include medication, physical therapy, steroid injections, and other interventions recommended by your health care team.

Certain conditions may impact the success and safety of SCS. Talk to your doctor if you have a bleeding or clotting disorders or are taking blood-thinning medications. Some types of stimulators can interfere with the function of cardiac pacemakers and defibrillators. Finally, you may need to proceed carefully if you have a condition that requires frequent MRIs (for example, multiple sclerosis), as some SCSs are not MRI compatible.

There are also practical considerations to having an SCS. Depending on the type of device, you may need to charge it regularly, control it with a handheld programmer, or wear an external power source around your waist. Stimulating your spinal cord while driving can cause a safety hazard, so you'll need to remember to turn off the device before you get behind the wheel. Eventually, you will probably need minor surgery to replace the stimulator's power source.

What to expect

SCS implantation is usually a two-step process. First, you'll go through a weeklong test phase in which the electrodes are placed so that the wires extend through the skin to a generator outside your body. The goal of the test is to reduce your pain by at least 50 percent and determine what stimulation "program" works best for you. If the trial is successful, your doctor will perform a second surgery to implant the generator beneath your skin.

Before implanting the electrodes, your doctor will numb the skin of your back with local anesthetic and give you a light sedative via IV. You'll need to be awake while the electrodes are placed and tested in order to let the doctor know when sensations occur and where, although recent studies suggest that electrode placement under general anesthesia tested with electrical stimulation monitoring may be equally effective.

To place the electrodes, the surgeon inserts a hollow introducer needle into the epidural space and threads the electrode through it. When the electrode is turned on, you should feel a mild tingling or numbness in the skin of your lower body. Ideally, your surgeon will place the electrodes so that they stimulate all the areas where you normally feel pain. Your doctor may try several different "programs" to see which one provides the most relief. Once the leads are in place and doing their job, you'll be given more local (or sometimes general) anesthetic so the leads can be anchored to your connective tissue. The procedure usually takes less than an hour.

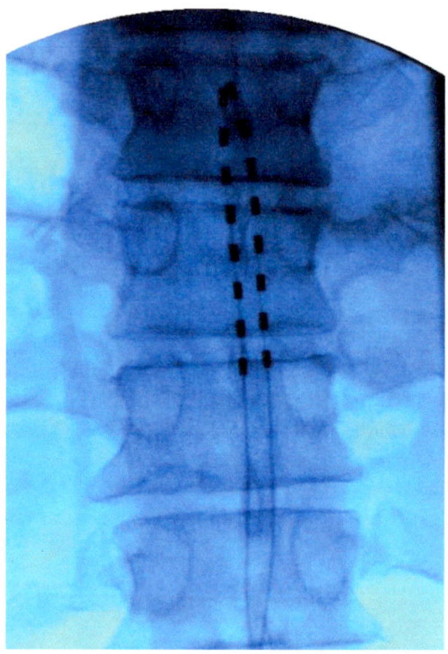

Figure 37: Image of a fifty-six-year-old woman who underwent laminectomy and spinal fusion from L4 through S1 four years ago. She developed severe leg pains two years after, but without evidence of a new herniation. Her MRI showed scar tissue around the nerves that exited through the previous surgery site. Epidural steroid injection therapy failed to help as did physical therapy. She underwent trial spinal spinal cord stimulation with one hundred percent relief of her leg symptoms. She also regained the ability to perform four primary activities that were limited by her pain (walking, housework, sleeping, and prolonged sitting).

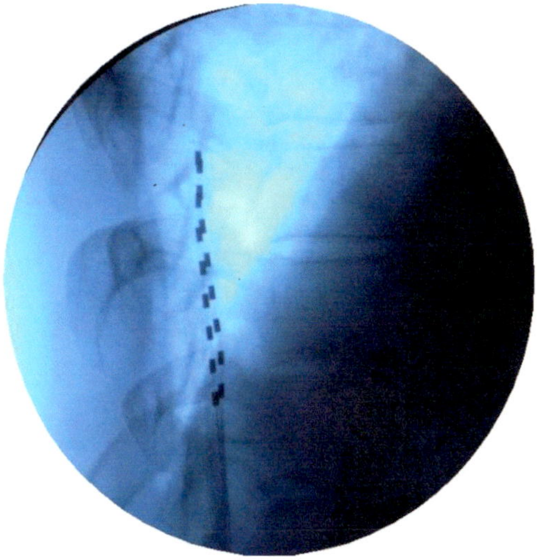

Figure 38: Lateral view of the same

After trial SCS implantation, your team will continue to experiment with different "programs" to find out which one works best for you during the postoperative period.

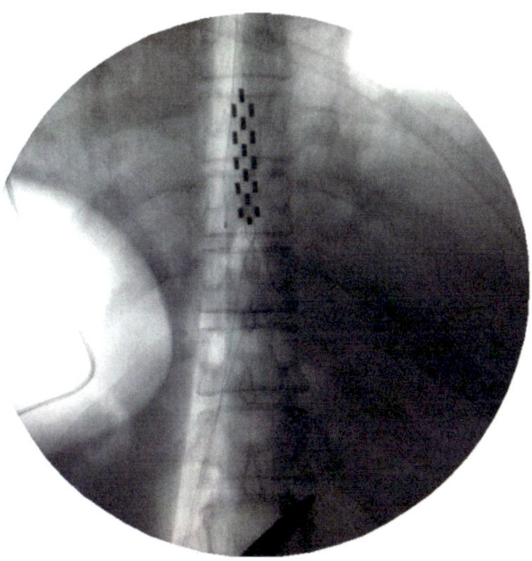

Figure 39: Permanent implantation provided sustained, long-term relief of her leg pain. Again, stimulation let her return to her everyday activities.

If the SCS trial is reasonably successful at relieving your symptoms, your doctor will schedule you for surgery to implant the permanent stimulator. At this time, the wires and generator will be placed under the skin of your abdomen or buttock. Some slack is left in the wires and generator "pocket" to allow for normal movement. This procedure may be performed under local or general anesthesia and may require an overnight hospital stay.

Risks and Side Effects

As noted above, SCS is quite safe, and serious neurological complications are rare. A systematic review involving over four thousand patients found that the most common complication is migration (movement) of the leads (13.5 percent of cases) and broken leads (7.6 percent of cases). These problems can usually be corrected by minor surgery.

Other potential risks include bleeding, infection, and accidental puncture of the dura (the tough sheathe which surrounds the spinal cord). The latter is usually not serious, but can cause headache after surgery.

Aftercare

During your SCS implantation trial, you should continue with your normal activities and medications unless directed otherwise by your doctor. Too many changes to your routine could mask the effects of stimulation and compromise the trial results. Your physician will prescribe oral antibiotics to prevent infection and (if needed) pain medications. You'll need to avoid twisting and bending your back for about a month, which may require some adjustments to your daily activities. However, light exercise like walking will promote healing.

Some people get worried when their pain doesn't go away completely during the trial period. Remember that total relief is rare during this time, and that a 50 percent decrease in pain intensity is considered a good result. Even after you receive your permanent stimulator, it may be a few weeks before you experience the full benefits.

John: Overcoming Setbacks

Eight months after his failed discectomy, John underwent a trial of spinal cord stimulation. The results were instant and dramatic. Just a few minutes after we activated the machine, his leg pain eased, and he was able to walk normally about the room. He estimated that the stimulator relieved his discomfort by at least 70 percent. These benefits continued throughout the weeklong trial period.

Today, John has a permanent stimulator and continues to show improvement. His pain is now 90 percent gone, and he only activates the device when needed. He was recently appointed the school's athletic director, and has seen several of his teams play in state-level championships. Best of all, he is able to be there for his family and friends when they need him (though he now stays off the roof).

Among friends and colleagues, he is outspoken about the importance of proper diagnosis before spine surgery. "Now that I pay more attention to these things, I'm surprised at how many people I know who are considering surgery, or have a loved one considering surgery," he says. "I wonder how many of them are really getting good advice from their doctors.

"When they ask me about it, I always try to drive home the importance of educating yourself and getting a second opinion. No lying, surgery is tough. You only want to go through that if you're likely to see real benefits."

Key Points

- A significant number of people continue to have some pain after back surgery. In a small percentage of cases, this discomfort is severe and disabling.
- Failed back surgery syndrome is caused by the formation of scar tissue at the site of a previous operation. If the scar is large enough, it can compress the nerve roots or invade the spinal canal.
- FBSS sometimes surfaces after the person goes months or even years without symptoms.
- Spinal cord stimulation is a safe and reversible treatment for FBSS pain.

This concludes our discussion of common back conditions and their treatments. In the final chapter, I'll offer some tips to get the most out of your back care—no matter what your diagnosis.

11

PARTING PRESCRIPTION: THREE TIPS TO GET THE MOST OUT OF YOUR TREATMENT

Congratulations. If you've read this far, you now understand the most common causes of low back pain and the available treatment options. More importantly, you know that there's hope for lasting relief—even if you've been told that your pain is normal or "all in your head."

So what do you do with your newfound knowledge? First and foremost, I hope you'll use it to take charge of your health care. Rather than relying blindly on your health care team for advice, treat them as expert partners who can guide your decision-making. Ask questions, propose next steps, and participate fully in the process. Never be afraid to disagree with suggestions you feel aren't in your best interest.

In this final chapter, I'll offer three tips that can help you avoid common pitfalls of the health care system. We'll also discuss what you can do outside the doctor's office to maximize your healing and well-being.

Prescription #1: Communicate with Your Health Care Team

Without a doubt, the culture of health care is changing. Economic realities now limit the amount of time that physicians spend with patients—particularly in primary care settings. On a brighter note, today's patients are far more informed and involved in their care, thanks in large part to advances like the Internet.

These changes impact the way patients and physicians interact. A few generations ago, doctors were viewed as all-knowing authority figures. By contrast, today's providers are more likely to talk through options with their patients and involve them in decision-making. This is why it's so important to be an expert in your own condition. The more you know about spine problems, the more you'll get out of these doctor-patients interactions.

You'll also have a better sense of your provider's limitations and know when it's time to seek a second opinion.

The following sections offer tips on communicating effectively with key members of your health care team.

Primary Care Providers

Your primary doctor is the first person you see when you have a concern about your health. This person is responsible for treating acute injuries and illnesses, managing chronic conditions, and delivering preventative care. Several types of professionals can fulfill this role, including general practice physicians, family physicians, internal medicine physicians, physician assistants, and nurse practitioners.

Low back pain is the fifth most common cause of primary care visits, according to the website of the American Academy of Family Physicians. However, as we've seen, many general practitioners are poorly equipped to diagnose and manage this condition. Too often, patients receive no treatment beyond conservative care and are referred for pain management if they don't improve within a few months.

Your primary provider doesn't need to have advanced training in spine disorders to be effective. However, he or she should:

- Listen and respond to your concerns and take them seriously.
- Practice evidence-based medicine that follows established clinical guidelines.
- Understand his or her own limitations and make appropriate referrals.
- Communicate effectively with specialists, therapists, and other members of your health care team.
- Assist in the coordination of your care.

The role your primary provider plays in your spine care will likely evolve over time. During the acute (early) phase, the most important task is to rule out "red flag" conditions such as cancer, infection, and autoimmune diseases. Assuming you have no signs of a serious underlying problem, your family doctor can recommend conservative interventions, prescribe needed medications, and monitor your condition.

Some primary care providers want to order elaborate diagnostic tests like MRIs during the acute phase—even when there are no indications of serious underlying illness. Such studies rarely reveal anything useful and can result in undue worry, inconvenience, and expense for the patient. If your provider suggests such a test, ask why. In many cases, your doctor is just trying to be thorough or cover certain bases. It's perfectly fine to suggest that you "wait and see" for the time being. You can always revisit imaging later if pain persists.

Furthermore, recent research suggests that imaging isn't a particularly useful tool in the primary care setting because providers don't necessarily know how to interpret the results. A 2012 Canadian study found that 44 percent of patients who underwent a lower back MRI in primary care were subsequently referred to orthopedic surgeons. However, only 6.5 percent of these people actually went on to have surgery. What's more, patients with relatively normal MRIs were just as likely to have an operation as those with multiple abnormalities. Researchers noted that because abnormal spinal MRI findings are common (occurring in as many as two-thirds of pain-free patients), primary care physicians might lack the clinical skill to discern between benign "wear and tear" and more serious structural abnormalities.

If your pain continues beyond four to six weeks, it's probably time to see a specialist for an in-depth diagnostic workup. Ideally, your primary care provider should remain involved by supporting and coordinating your care. Practices that excel in this role can help facilitate communication between providers, manage your records, and spot errors and redundancies. This ensures your safety and can often save you money and hassle as well.

Interventionists

Interventional spine pain specialists use minimally invasive procedures to diagnose and treat painful spine conditions. Common examples include spinal nerve blocks, disc stimulation, radiofrequency denervation, epidural steroid injections, and minimally invasive surgeries. Increasingly, these interventions represent a safer alternative to traditional surgery.

Interventional spine medicine is a relatively new field, and primary care physicians are usually less familiar with it than with surgery. For this reason, you may need to specifically request a referral to an interventionist. In some areas, relatively few physicians specialize in interventional spine care, so finding a good one may require some research (and possibly travel).

Seek out the most experienced interventionist you can find. At present, the American Board of Medical Specialties does not offer certification in interventional medicine. However, your choice should ideally be board-certified in a related specialty (most commonly surgery, pain management, or physical medicine). He or she should also have completed fellowship-level training in this specialty.

Often, interventionists work closely with physical medicine and rehabilitation physicians (also called physiatrists), and many are board-certified in this specialty. Physiatrists are trained to design effective therapy programs that can complement your interventional care and improve your overall function and conditioning.

Back Surgeons

Because approximately 80 to 90 percent of spine pain cases can be treated without surgery, referral for surgical evaluations is rarely (if ever) necessary during the acute phase. This is frequently done, however, because of lingering misconceptions.

Until relatively recently, interventional spine pain physicians simply did not exist. Surgery was therefore the only option when conservative therapy failed. When completing our primary care rotations in medical school and in medical internship, were taught to refer back pain patients to a surgeon as a matter of course.

Fortunately, times have changed. Today's patients have access to a growing variety of minimally invasive treatments. It is most appropriate to hold off on making a surgical referral unless the patient has signs of a serious condition, including:

- Progressive extremity weakness
- Bowel or bladder dysfunction
- Spine instability
- Fracture
- Tumors

So when should you consider seeing a surgeon? Aside from above, there are no clear cut guidelines for this. If your leg pain is debilitating , and doesn't respond to at least six months of aggressive conservative therapy including appropriately performed epidural steroid injection procedures with appropriate physician directed therapeutic exercises, it may be time to revisit the idea. Leg pain, which is often due to nerve compression, is somewhat more responsive to surgical treatment than mechanical pain.

Before taking the surgical route, it's generally a good idea to thoroughly review your case with the best spine specialist you can find. Get at least more than one opinion. How confident are they with your diagnosis? Are less aggressive treatments available? Also, consider the fact that back pain tends to wax and wane depending on your activity level. Would you be willing to modify your lifestyle to avoid the risks of surgery? All of these questions should be answered to your satisfaction before a decision to pursue surgery is made.

Prescription #2: Act Sooner Rather than Later

When back pain first flares up, trying a couple months of conservative care makes sense. However, living too long with debilitating pain can push both your body and mind past the breaking point, as happened to Mr. Jones in Chapter 2.

Research strongly suggests that chronic back pain is most responsive to treatment during its early months before physical deterioration, depression, relationship problems, and financial difficulties take their toll on the patient. However, many primary care physicians make the mistake of prolonging conservative care long past the point of reason.

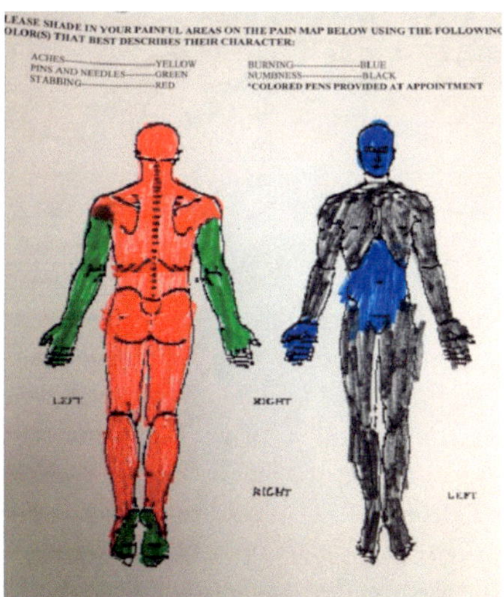

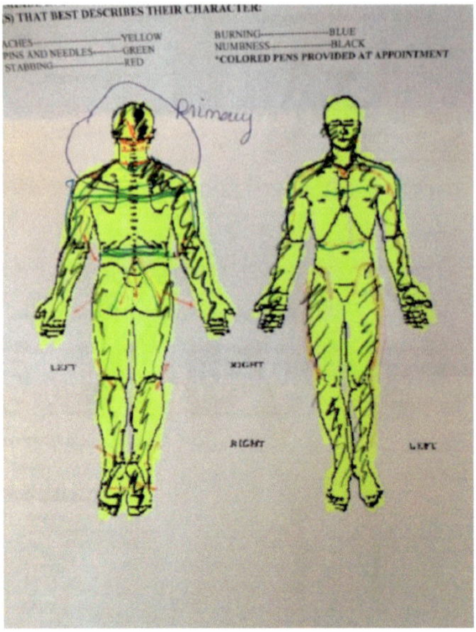

Pain diagrams created by patients with chronic back pain. In each person, the pain began as a localized problem (e.g., back or leg pain). Over time, these patients developed depression, anxiety, and whole-body pain until they were essentially "hurting all over." Early, diagnosis-directed treatment is critical to prevent long-term emotional consequences.

Why does this happen so often? As you'll recall from Chapter 1, many physicians have been erroneously taught that mostly all of low back pain patients recover within three months, with or without treatment and many patients with back pain are subject to nonspecific symptomatic treatment.

This myth dates back to a flawed 1966 study, the results of which were widely reported in the medical world.

Emerging evidence suggests that this status quo is not only based on flawed assumptions, it may actually harm some patients. A 2012 survey of five hundred eighty-nine people seeking treatment for low back pain found that 73 percent had experienced a recurrence at some point after their first episode. What's more, 66 percent reported that their episodes were worsening in at least one of five key domains. By contrast, only 4 percent rated their latest recurrence as less severe or the same as their original episode. These findings suggest that contrary to popular belief, low back pain:

- Is not always a harmless condition
- Can recur frequently
- Tends to worsen with each recurrence
- May eventually evolve into constant (chronic) pain

In response to the above paper, a group of concerned practitioners from the Hospital for Special Surgery in New York wrote a letter to the editor of Spine calling for additional research on the subject. They felt that it was important to understand which patients were prone to recurrent, worsening low back pain, as these people represented an at-risk population. "This group cannot be treated with benign neglect," the authors wrote. "Instead they require timely interventions and comprehensive rehabilitation to resolve pain, restore function, and prevent recurrences of LBP."

Bottom line: letting back pain go untreated for too long can be hazardous to your health. If discomfort persists beyond three months, request a referral to a specialist so you can obtain a definitive diagnosis and explore the full range of treatment options.

Prescription #3: Maintain a Healthy Lifestyle

Chronic and preventable illnesses like obesity, diabetes, heart disease, and high blood pressure are on the rise and currently account for 75 percent of American health care spending. Common sense suggests that being overweight puts additional strain on your spine. So, you may wonder, why have I waited until the very end of the book to discuss the importance of a healthy lifestyle?

There are three reasons. First, when it comes to back pain, some risk factors are clearly out of your control. Numerous studies have linked sciatica, disc herniation, and disc degeneration to genetic factors—and even identified certain genes responsible. For example, the gene COL9A1 synthesizes collagen IX, a protein and important building block of cartilage. In some people, this gene expresses by producing an alternate type of protein, which results in less and weaker cartilage throughout the body. People with this gene type (allele) appear to be more prone to osteoarthritis—and to experience it at an earlier age. In addition, certain spine conditions, notably ankylosing spondylitis and inflammatory arthritis, appear to have a strong genetic component.

Second, the body of research linking certain lifestyle factors with low back pain is incomplete. The evidence we do have tends to be in the form of correlations. In other words, when we see a lot of X, we also tend to see a lot of Y. But due to limitations of the study design, we can't say for sure that X is causing Y.

Here's a real life example. A recent study followed two hundred fifty people with chronic low back pain and z-joint arthritis for one year. At the end of the study, people with elevated blood sugar were also found to have more pain-related disability.

Based on the study, can we say that high blood sugar causes persistent, disabling low back pain? Well, not exactly. To say that, we would need a more sophisticated research design that allowed for in-depth statistical analysis. We might in fact find out the opposite—that back pain causes high blood sugar (perhaps because people are less active when they're in chronic pain).

That being said, we do know from previous research that excess blood glucose has a number of adverse effects on the body that could potentially contribute to back pain. For example, high blood sugar can interfere with bone metabolism, which might lead to inflammation of the z-joints. There's also evidence that excess sugar can increase pain sensitivity within connective tissue. And finally, chronic excess sugar in the form of diabetes contributes to atherosclerosis, which reduces blood flow to the spine and has been shown to accelerate disc and joint degeneration.

Bottom line: while we can't yet make a direct link between blood sugar and spine pain, that's probably the way to bet. Back pain patients who also have prediabetes or diabetes certainly have nothing to lose and everything to gain by managing their condition. And primary care physicians would be wise to screen new back pain patients for high blood sugar.

This brings us to my third caveat when it comes to lifestyle factors: lack of scientific evidence hasn't stopped some professionals from using them as metaphorical clubs to beat their patients. This is particularly unfortunate in the case of overweight people, who are told that shedding a few pounds will fix everything.

As we'll see in a moment, this argument is demonstrably accurate for people who happen to be morbidly obese. However, if we're just talking about a few extra pounds, weight may actually have a protective effect. A study involving male identical twins of differing sizes found that the spines of the heavier twins actually showed fewer degenerative changes. Conversely, people with very slight builds are prone to osteoporosis, which is a serious risk factor for spine problems.

No one really understands how excess weight impacts the spine. The relationship is likely a complicated one involving interplay of mechanical and metabolic factors. Existing research suggests that people who are obese (defined as having a body mass index of 30 or more) do appear to be at increased risk for developing chronic low back pain. A 2004 Norwegian study analyzed the results of two health surveys carried out a decade apart. The team found that obese men were 34 percent more likely to develop chronic low back pain over that period than those with a BMI under 25. For women, obesity elevated the risk by 22 percent. Sufficient data was available to control for lifestyle factors such as tobacco use, inactivity, and weight gain. None of these seemed to impact the relationship between obesity and chronic back pain.

Research also suggests that losing weight can have a beneficial effect on back pain. A study published in 2013 followed a group of very obese back pain patients (BMI 40 or greater) for a year after bariatric surgery. Not only did the patients lose a significant amount of weight, their lumbar disc heights actually increased. They also reported significantly less low back pain and leg pain one year after surgery.

Bottom line: while the relationship between back pain and a healthy lifestyle isn't clear-cut, you have nothing to lose by making reasonable changes to your diet and habits. Remember, even small adjustment can make a difference. Pain is already taking up a lot of your energy, so keep your goals small and realistic.

Some practical suggestions:

- Ask your doctor for advice. A good primary care physician is your best ally when it comes to lifestyle changes like losing weight, quitting smoking, or controlling your diabetes.
- Make sure you are up-to-date on your recommended health screenings. Chronic conditions like high blood pressure and diabetes often have no symptoms.
- If you're overweight, losing just ten to fifteen pounds can have a significant effect on your blood sugar, according to the American Diabetes Association. Start by making small but positive changes to your diet.
- Stay as active as your back pain will allow. Walking for thirty minutes a day on most days will burn calories and help you achieve a basic level of fitness. If you can't do thirty minutes at

once, try breaking your workout into two fifteen-minute sessions. Physical therapy and aqua therapy also provide good workouts. Some people report that yoga not only improves their fitness but also temporarily eases their pain.

- Smoking is associated with poor outcomes for back pain patients, particularly those who undergo surgery. Your doctor can prescribe medications that make quitting easier.
- Chronic pain can be a depressing, isolating experience, so pay attention to your emotional health. Your family members may also need extra support during this time. Many health systems and community organizations provide counseling, support groups, and educational programs for people impacted by chronic pain.

Remember, you don't have to do everything on your own. If you're struggling with change, consider consulting a dietitian, behavioral therapist, personal trainer, or other expert. Your doctor can often provide recommendations.

Parting Words

Well, it's happened. We've come to the end. I hope this little handbook has left you enlightened, excited, and above all hopeful about the many possibilities available to people living with chronic low back pain.

This book is intended to provide a comprehensive overview of some common spine problems. That being said, it is neither a Bible nor a textbook on the subject. I urge you to continue your education through further reading and discussions with your physician. Be that bold, inquisitive person who's always asking questions. Make a point of becoming a leading expert on your own condition.

Above all, advocate for yourself. Refuse to accept "benign neglect" and canned answers to your questions. Don't let any person—especially a health care professional—sentence you to a lifetime of pain and disability. Seek out the best care and most experienced practitioners available. Be relentless in your search for answers.

And remember:
"Nothing happens until something moves."

- Albert Einstein

ENDNOTES

Image Credits

The folowing images were adapted with permission granted from Elsevier: figure 2, figure 4, figure 6, figure 7, figure 12, figure 27. Original images from CLINICAL AND RADIOLOGICAL ANATOMY OF THE LUMBAR SPINE 5/E, 9780702043420, 2012, Bogduk.

Chapter 1

25 percent of Americans have at least one day of low back pain in any three month period: "Handout on Health: Back Pain," National Institute of Arthritis, Musculoskeletal and Skin Diseases, accessed January 23, 2013, http://www.niams.nih.gov/health_info/Back_Pain/default.asp.

Lifetime prevalence of low back pain as high as 80 percent: D.I. Rubin, "Epidemiology and Risk Factors for Spine Pain," Neurology Clinics 2 (2007): 353.

Back pain is the second most common cause of disability in adults: Centers for Disease Control, "Prevalence of Disabilities and Associated Health Conditions Among Adults—United States, 1999," Journal of the American Medical Association 12 (2001): 1571-2.

Annual costs of low back pain exceed $100 billion: J.N. Katz, "Lumbar Disc Disorders and Low-Back Pain: Socioeconomic Factors and Consequences," Journal of Bone & Joint Surgery 2S (2006): 21.

North Carolina study suggests sharp rise in the incidence of low back pain: J.K. Freburger et al., "The Rising Prevalence of Chronic Low Back Pain," Archives of Internal Medicine 3 (2009): 251.

Japanese study points to occupational and psychosocial risk factors: K. Matsudaira et al., "Potential Risk Factors for New Onset of Back Pain Disability in Japanese Workers," Spine 15 (2012): 1324-33.

Ninety percent of low back pain patients return to work within three months: Robert L. Bratton, "Assessment and Management for Acute Low Back Pain," American Family Physician 8: 2299.

One-year recurrence rate of 50 to 80 percent for acute low back pain: "Clinical Evidence Concise: Acute Low Back Pain," American Academy of Family Physicians, accessed March 22, 2013, http://www.aafp.org/afp/2006/0901/p803.html.

Flawed 1966 study leads many physicians to delay intervention: Discussed in Ronald Donelson, Greg McIntosh, and Hamilton Hall, "Is It Time to Rethink the Typical Course of Low Back Pain?" Physical Medicine and Rehabilitation 6 (2012): 394-401. We'll revisit this study and new research contradicting its findings in Chapter 11.

Spinal injuries missed by MRI, verified in cadaver study: Nikolai Bogduk, "On Cervical Zygapophysial Joint Pain After Whiplash," Spine 25S (2011): 194-99.

Chapter 3

Sixty percent of back pain patients feel better within a week: Robert L. Bratton, "Assessment and Management for Acute Low Back Pain," American Family Physician 8: 2299.

Clinical guidelines note contradictory scientific evidence: Roger Chou et al., "Diagnosis and Treatment of Low Back Pain: A Joint Clinical Practice Guideline from the American College of Physicians and the American Pain Society," Annals of Internal Medicine 7 (2007): 479.

Cochrane Review found better outcomes for patients who stayed active: Kare B. Hagen et al., "The Updated Cochrane Review of Bed Rest for Low Back Pain and Sciatica," Spine 5 (2005): 542-46.

American College of Physicians recommends against prolonged bed rest: This and all other recommendations attributed in-text to the ACP are drawn from Chou et al., "Diagnosis and Treatment," 478-491.

Bed rest had no effect on sciatica: Hagen et al., "Updated Cochrane Review."

NSAIDs may be no more effective than acetaminophen: Pepijn D. D. M. Roelofs et al., "Anti-inflammatory Drugs for Low Back Pain: An Updated Cochrane Review," Spine 16 (2008): 1766-74.

COX-2 inhibitors may increase the risk of serious cardiovascular side effects: Roelofs et al., "Anti-inflammatory Drugs."

Systematic review found muscle relaxants are generally effective for low back pain, but prone to side effects: Maurits van Tulder et al., "Muscle Relaxants for Nonspecific Low Back Pain: A Systematic Review Within the Framework of the Cochrane Collaboration," Spine 17 (2003): 1978-92.

Opioid therapy achieved a thirty percent reduction in average pain intensity: Eija Kalso et al., "Opioids in Chronic Non-Cancer Pain: Systematic Review of Efficacy and Safety," Pain 3 (2004): 372-80.

Weaker opioids no more effective than NSAIDs at relieving back pain: Andrea D. Furlan et al., "Opioids for Chronic Noncancer Pain: A Meta-Analysis of Effectiveness and Side Effects," Canadian Medical Association Journal 11 (2006): 1589-94.

High rate of substance abuse among participants in opioid drug trials: Bridget A. Martell et al., "Systematic Review: Opioid Treatment for Chronic Back Pain: Prevalence, Efficacy, and Association with Addiction," Annals of Internal Medicine 2 (2007) 116-27.

Eighty percent of opioid trial participants experienced side effects: Kalso et al., "Opioids in Chronic Non-Cancer Pain."

Opioids cause significantly more nausea and constipation than other painkillers: Furlan et al., "Opioids for Chronic Non-Cancer Pain."

Gabapentin relieves leg pain (but not associated back pain) in 2001 trial: Gary McCleane, "Does Gabapentin Have an Analgesic Effect on Background, Movement and Referred Pain? A Randomised, Double-Blind, Placebo Controlled Study," The Pain Clinic 2 (2001): 103-107.

Sciatica patients show functional improvement after gabapentin therapy: Kadir Yildirim et al., "The Effectiveness of Gabapentin in Patients with Chronic Radiculopathy," The Pain Clinic 3 (2003): 213-218.

Depression and pain may share biological pathways: Matthew J. Bair et al., "Depression and Pain Comorbidity: A Literature Review," Archives of Internal Medicine 20 (2003): 2433-45.

Two systematic reviews independently confirm the effectiveness of tricyclic antidepressant therapy for back pain: Stephen M. Salerno, Robert Browning, and Jeffrey L. Jackson, "The Effect of Antidepressant Treatment on Chronic Back Pain: A Meta-Analysis," Archives of Internal Medicine 1 (2002): 19-24, and Thomas O. Staiger et al., "Systematic Review of Antidepressants in the Treatment of Chronic Low Back Pain," Spine 22 (2003): 2540-45.

SSRIs have no direct therapeutic effect on back pain: Staiger et al., "Review of Antidepressant Treatment."

Cochrane Review team finds poor-quality evidence on the effectiveness of herbal medicines: Joel J. Gagnier et al., "Herbal Medicine for Low Back Pain," Cochrane Database of Systematic Reviews 2 (2006): CD004504.

Multiple Cochrane Reviews conclude that spinal manipulative therapy has no significant benefits over other conservative treatments: Willem J. Assendelft et al., "Spinal Manipulative Therapy for Low Back Pain. A Meta-Analysis of Effectiveness Relative to Other Therapies," Annals of Internal Medicine 11 (2003): 871-81, and Sidney M. Rubinstein et al., "Spinal Manipulative Therapy for Chronic Low-Back Pain: An Update of a Cochrane Review," Spine 13 (2011): E825-46. It's worth noting that the lead author in the 2011 review is a chiropractor.

Exercise may actually prolong acute low back pain: Antti Malmivaara et al., "The Treatment of Acute Low Back Pain—Bed Rest, Exercises, or Ordinary Activity?" New England Journal of Medicine 6 (1995): 351.

Systematic review shows no benefits for exercise during acute stage of back pain: Maurits van Tulder et al., "Exercise Therapy for Low Back Pain: A Systematic Review Within the Framework of the Cochrane Collaboration Back Review Group," Spine 21 (2000): 2784-96.

Tailored, supervised exercise programs benefit patients with acute low back pain: Jill A. Hayden, Maurits W. van Tulder, and George Tomlinson, "Systematic Review: Strategies for Using Exercise Therapy to

Improve Outcomes in Chronic Low Back Pain," Annals of Internal Medicine 9 (2005): 776-85.

More rigorous trials of TENS needed: Amole Khadilkar et al., "Transcutaneous Electrical Nerve Stimulation for the Treatment of Chronic Low Back Pain: A Systematic Review," Spine 23 (2005): 2657-66.

Cochrane Review finds no evidence for traction's effectiveness: Judy A. Clarke et al., "Traction for Low Back Pain With or Without Sciatica: An Updated Systematic Review Within the Framework of the Cochrane Collaboration," Spine 14, (2007): 1591–99.

Thirty-eight percent of Americans use alternative medicine: "What Is Complementary and Alternative Medicine?" National Center for Complimentary and Alternative Medicine, accessed March 22, 2013, http://nccam.nih.gov/health/whatiscam.

Acupuncture and dry-needling show promise in the treatment of back pain: Andrea D. Furlan et al., "Acupuncture and Dry-Needling for Low Back Pain: An Updated Systematic Review Within the Framework of the Cochrane Collaboration," Spine 8 (2005): 944-63, and Eric Manheimer et al., "A Meta-Analysis: Acupuncture for Low Back Pain," Annals of Internal Medicine 8 (2005): 651-63.

Massage shows promise in the treatment of chronic low back pain: Andrea D. Furlan et al., "Massage for Low-Back Pain: A Systematic Review Within the Framework of the Cochrane Collaboration Back Review Group," Spine 17 (2002): 1896-910.

Psychological problems are a consequence and not a cause of pain in whiplash patients: Linda J. Carroll, J. David Cassidy J, and Pierre Cote, "Frequency, Timing, and Course Of Depressive Symptomatology after Whiplash," Spine 16 (2006): E551-56, and Bogdan P. Radanov, "Course of Psychological Variables in Whiplash Injury—A 2-Year Follow-Up with Age, Gender and Education Pair-Matched Patients," Pain 3 (1996): 429-434.

Psychological interventions can lead to better outcomes for back pain patients: Benson M. Hoffman et al., "Meta-Analysis of Psychological Interventions for Chronic Low Back Pain," Health Psychology 1 (2007): 1-9.

Chapter 4

No correlation between disc degeneration and pain: Research on the subject is summarized by Paul E. Verrills, Nikolai Bogduk, and David G. Vivian, "Diagnostic Imaging of Lumbosacral Disc Disruption," in iSpine: Evidence-Based Interventional Spine Care, ed. Michael DePalma, (New York: Demos Medical Publishing, 2011), 36-43.

Disc degeneration is very common in people who are asymptomatic: Evidence, including results of a 1997 systematic review, are summarized by Nikolai Bogduk in "Degenerative Joint Disease of the Spine," Radiologic Clinics of North America 4 (2012): 613-628.

Bogduk suggests physicians refer to disc degeneration as "normal age changes": Bogduk, "Degenerative Joint Disease," 625. The author, a preeminent researcher in the field of spine pain, calls the term degenerative "unnecessary and emotive." He even goes so far as to say that it can be "expunged from the radiologic lexicon."

Disc innervation of the inner annulus and nucleus relatively common: A.J. Freemont et al., "Nerve Ingrowth into Diseased Intervertebral Disc in Chronic Back Pain," Lancet 350 (1997): 178-81.

Graded severity of IDD: Grades are listed according to the Dallas Discogram Scale, first described by Barton L. Sachs et al., "Dallas Discogram Description: A New Classification of CT/Discography in Low-Back Disorders," Spine 3 (1987): 287–94.

Endplates can fail after as few as one hundred repetitions: Numbers and forces are calculated based on the results of a pair of studies: Y.K. Liu et al., "Fatigue Response of Lumbar Intervertebral Joints under Axial Cyclic Loading," Spine 8 (1983): 857-65; and T.H. Hansson, T.S. Keller, and D.M. Spengler, "Mechanical Behaviour of the Human Lumbar Spine. II. Fatigue Strength During Dynamic Compressive Loading," Journal of Orthopaedic Research 4 (1987):479–87.

Holt study finds high false-positive rates for discography: Earl P. Holt, "The Question Of Lumbar Discography," Journal of Bone and Joint Surgery 4 (1968): 720-726. In addition to failing to control for injection pressures, Holt tested his theory on asymptomatic patients who, by definition, cannot report "reproduced" pain. The true number of positives (false or otherwise) produced by this method would therefore be zero.

Derby's disc stimulation findings contradict Holt's—no pain in healthy subjects at recommended pressure thresholds: Richard Derby et al., "Comparison of Discographic Findings in Asymptomatic Subject Discs and the Negative Discs of Chronic LBP Patients: Can Discography Distinguish Asymptomatic Discs Among Morphologically Abnormal Discs?" Spine 4 (2005): 389-394. During the study, researchers adhered strictly to the recommended protocols of the International Spine Intervention Society (ISIS).

Study involving 4,319 patients finds 1-percent false positive rate for discography: Kevin Pauza, Susan Howell, and Paul Dreyfuss, "A Randomized, Placebo Controlled Trial of Intradiscal Electrothermal Therapy for the Treatment of Discogenic Low Back Pain," Spine 4 (2004): 27-35. The study was recognized as a North American Spine Society Outstanding Paper of 2003.

Carragee finds evidences of long-term disc problems in discography patients: Eugene J. Carragee et al., "Can Discography Cause Long-Term Back Symptoms in Previously Asymptomatic Patients?" Spine 14 (2000): 1803-1808. Carragee was also lead author on several papers that purported to find a high false-positive rate for discography.

2012 study by Derby and colleagues supports FAD's effectiveness: Richard Derby et al., "Comparison of Four Different Analgesic Discogram Protocols Comparing the Incidence of Reported Pain Relief Following Local Anesthetic Injection into Concordantly Painful Lumbar Intervertebral Discs," Pain Medicine 12 (2012): 1547-1553.

Preliminary evidence on epidural steroid injection efficacy: Jung Hwan Lee, Ju Ha An, and Sang-Ho Lee, "Comparison of the Effectiveness of Interlaminar and Bilateral Transforaminal Epidural Steroid Injections in Treatment of Patients with Lumbosacral Disc Herniation and Spinal Stenosis," Clinical Journal of Pain Management 3 (2009): 206-10.

Intradiscal methylene blue injection provides significant relief in 90 percent of participants: Baogan Peng et al., "Intradiscal Methylene Blue Injection for the Treatment of Chronic Discogenic Low Back Pain," European Spine Journal 1 (2007): 33-38.

Korean study finds fewer long-term benefits for methylene blue injection: S.H. Kim et al., "Effect of Intradiscal Methylene Blue Injection for the Chronic Discogenic Low Back Pain: One Year Prospective Follow-up Study," Annals of Physical and Rehabilitation Medicine 5 (2012): 657-64.

IDET provides statistically significant relief in carefully selected patient groups: Pauza et al., "Placebo Controlled Trial."

Biologic approaches: Information on evidence to date was drawn from two summaries: Michael DePalma, "Biologic Treatments for Discogenic Low Back Pain," SpineLine March/April (2012): 19-26; and Rajeev K. Patel, "Intradiscal Biologic Agents for Lumbosacral Internal Disc Disruption," in iSpine: Evidence-Based Interventional Spine Care, ed. Michael DePalma (New York: Demos Medical Publishing, 2011), 74-78.

Biostat System shows promise: 2013 North American Spine Society New Spine Technology Conference, Kevin Pauza presentation.

Chapter 5

Marvin's case study:.As a long-haul trucker, Marvin in one of the occupations most at risk for back problems, along with nurses, teachers, construction workers, professional movers, firefighters, and those who spend long hours at their computers each day.

Spinal x-rays of as many as 60 percent of twenty-somethings show arthritic changes: Jason D. Eubanks et al., "Prevalence of Lumbar Facet Arthrosis and Its Relationship to Age, Sex, and Race: An Anatomic Study of Cadaveric Specimens," Spine 19 (2007): 2058-62.

Kaplan study supports MBB's effectiveness as a diagnostic tool: Michael Kaplan et al., "The Ability of Lumbar Medial Branch Blocks to Anesthetize the Zygapophysial Joint. A Physiologic Challenge," Spine 17 (1998): 1847-52.

Radiofrequency ablation provides effective but temporary relief: Jerome Schofferman and Garrett Kine, "Effectiveness of Repeated Radiofrequency Neurotomy for Lumbar Facet Pain," Spine 21 (2004): 2471-73.

Problems with existing systematic reviews on RFN efficacy: Nikolai Bogduk, Paul Dreyfuss, and Jayantilal Govind, "A Narrative Review of Lumbar Branch Neurotomy for the Treatment of Lower Back Pain," Pain Medicine 6 (2009): 1035-1045.

Chapter 6

SI joint pain commonly coexists with other back conditions: T.N. Bernard and William H. Kirkaldy-Willis, "Recognizing Specific Characteristics of Non-Specific Low Back Pain," Clinical Orthopaedics and Related Research 217 (1987): 266-280.

Prevalence of SI joint pain increases with age: Michael J. DePalma, Jessica M. Ketchum, and Thomas Saullo, "What is the source of chronic low back pain and does age play a role?" Pain Medicine, 12 (2): 224-233.

Increased motion and pressure on SI joints after lumbar spinal fusion: Alexander A. Ivanov et al., "Lumbar fusion leads to increases in angular motion and stress across sacroiliac joint: a finite element study," Spine 5 (2009): E162-69.

Forty percent of failed back surgery syndrome patients appear to have SI involvement: Derived from a number of studies, including J.Y. Maigne and C.A. Planchon, "Sacroiliac Joint Pain after Lumbar Fusion. A Study with Anesthetic Blocks," European Spine Journal 7 (2005): 654-58, and Michael J. DePalma, Jessica M. Ketchum, and Thomas R. Saullo, "Etiology of Chronic Low Back Pain in Patients Having Undergone Lumbar Fusion," Pain Medicine 5 (2011): 732-39. These papers reported prevalences of 35 and 42 percent respectively.

Specific physical examination findings correlate with diagnostic block results: M. Laslett et al., "Diagnosing Painful Sacroiliac Joints: A Validity Study of a Mckenzie Evaluation and Sacroiliac Provocation Tests," Australian Journal of Physiotherapy 49 (2003): 89-97

High false positive rates for lateral branch block: Reports resulted by J.Y. Maigne, A. Aivalikilis, and Fabrice Pfefer, "Results of Sacroiliac Joint Double Block and Value of Sacroiliac Pain Provocation Tests in 54 Patients with Low Back Pain," Spine 16 (1996): 1889-92.

Seventy percent efficacy for LBB with multi-site, multi-depth injections: P. Dreyfuss, T. Henning, N. Malladi, B. Goldstein, and Nikolai Bogduk, "The ability of multi-site, multi-depth sacral lateral branch blocks to anesthetize the sacroiliac joint complex," Pain Medicine 4 (2009): 679-88.

Austrian study on cooled RFN efficacy: Wolfgang Stelzer et al., "Use of Cooled Radiofrequency Lateral Branch Neurotomy for the Treatment of Sacroiliac Joint-Mediated Low Back Pain: A Large Case Series," Pain Medicine 14 (2013): 29-35.

Efficacy of intra-articular approaches to neurotomy: F.M. Ferrante, et al., "Radiofrequency Sacroiliac Joint Denvervation for Sacroiliac Joint Syndrome," Regional Anesthesia and Pain Medicine 2 (2001): 137-142.

Chapter 7

Disc herniation prevalence is 1 to 3 percent: "Lumbar Disc Herniation," http://bestpractice.bmj.com/best-practice/evidence/background/1118.html, accessed March 12, 2013.

Chemical radiculitis animal model: Jason M. Cuellar et al., "Cytokine Expression in the Epidural Space," Spine 1 (2012): 17-23.

Forty percent of patients with pain below the knee are later diagnosed with radiculopathy: S. Haldeman, M. Shouka, and S. Robboy, "Computed Tomography, Electrodiagnostic and Clinical Findings in Chronic Workers' Compensation Patients With Back and Leg Pain," Spine 3 (1995): 318-27.

Seventy percent of patients with radiculopathy show some neurologic changes: Phillip Tasca, "An Algorithmic Approach to Lumbosacral Radiculopathy," in iSpine: Evidence-Based Interventional Spine Care, ed. Michael DePalma (New York: Demos Medical Publishing, 2011), 171.

Positive straight leg test correlates with disc herniation radiculopathy: W.R. Hudgins, "The Crossed Straight-Leg Raising Test: A Diagnostic Sign of Herniated Disc," Journal of Occupational Medicine 6 (1979): 407-08, and Lawrence F. Supik and Michael J. Broom, "Sciatic Tension Signs and Lumbar Disc Herniation," Spine 9 (1994): 1066-69. Authors report a specificity of 97 percent and 90 percent respectively.

Spinal nerve block findings confirmed by later surgery: D. Stanley et al., "A Prospective Study of Nerve Root Infiltration in the Diagnosis of Sciatica—A Comparison with Radiculography, Computer Tomography, and Operative Findings," Spine 6 (1990): 540-43. These findings supported the conclusions of several earlier studies dating back to the 1970s.

Systematic review of transforaminal epidural steroid injections for radicular pain: John MacVicar et al., "The Effectiveness of Lumbar Transforaminal Injection of Steroids: A Comprehensive Review with Systematic Analysis of the Published Data," Pain Medicine 14 (2013): 14-28.

Chapter 8

Most common disorder in older people: "Spinal stenosis," http://emedicine.medscape.com/article/1913265-overview#a0156, accessed March 1, 2013.

Relationship between spinal stenosis and lifestyle related illness: Kazuhide Uesugi et al., "Relationship Between Lumbar Spinal Stenosis and Lifestyle-Related Disorders: A Cross-Sectional Multi-Center Observational Study," Spine Publish Ahead of Print (2013) doi:10.1097/BRS.0b013e31828a2517.

Spinal stenosis is frequently an improving syndrome (Michigan Spinal Stenosis Study): Andrew J. Haig et al., "Predictors of Pain and Function in Persons with Spinal Stenosis, Low Back Pain, and No Back Pain," Spine 25 (2006): 2950-57.

Difficulty of differentiating co-morbid hip arthritis and spinal stenosis: Junya Saito et al., "Difficulty of Diagnosing the Origin of Lower Leg Pain in Patients with Both Lumbar Spinal Stenosis and Hip Joint Osteoarthritis," Spine 25 (2012): 2089-93.

Diagnostic validity of electrodiagnosis tests: Haig et al., "Predictors of Pain," 2956.

Sixty-nine percent of surgeons consider ESI a front-line treatment: Bryan Lebude et al., "Clinical Survey: Patterns of Utilization of Lumbar Epidural Steroid Injections by a Cohort of Spinal Surgeons," PM&R 1 (2009): 329-34.

Limited systematic review of epidural spinal injections for radicular lumbar pain: L. Manchikanti et al., "Effectiveness of Therapeutic Lumbar Transforaminal Epidural Injections in Managing Lumbar Spine Pain," Pain Physician 3 (2012): E199-245.

Worse outcomes in patients treated with epidural steroid injections: Kris Radcliff et al., "Epidural Steroid Injections Are Associated With Less Improvement in Patients With Lumbar Spinal Stenosis: A Subgroup Analysis of the Spine Patient Outcomes Research Trial," Spine 4 (2013): 279-91.

Systematic review of IPSs suggests mechanical benefits, advantages over conservative therapy: Syed M. R. Kabir et al., "Lumbar Interspinous Spacers: A Systematic Review of Clinical and Biomechanical Evidence," Spine 25 (2010): E1499-1506.

X-STOP FDA approval study showed significant improvements: Discussed in relation to later studies in Kabir et al, "Lumbar Interspinous Spacers," E1501-2.

Potential conflict of interest during X-STOP's FDA study: Discussed in David H. Kim et. al., "Occult Spinous Process Fractures Associated with Interspinous Process Spacers," Spine 16 (2011): E1085.

X-STOP cost-effectiveness study: Grant Skidmore et al., "Cost-Effectiveness of the X-STOP Interspinous Spacer for Lumbar Spinal Stenosis: A Comparison with Conservative Care and Laminectomy," Spine 5 (2011): E346-356.

Fracture rates for IPSs higher than previous reported: Kim et al., "Occult Spinous Process Fractures," E1080-85.

Complication rates for X-STOP: X-STOP Interspinous Process Decompression System, application number P040001, FDA approval November 21, 2005.

Cleveland Clinic mild trial: N. Mekhail et al., "Long-Term Results of Percutaneous Lumbar Decompression mild for Spinal Stenosis," Pain Practice 3 (2012): 184-93.

2012 systematic safety review of mild: Robert M. Levy and Timothy R. Deer, "Systematic Safety Review and Meta-Analysis of Procedural

Experience Using Percutaneous Access to Treat Symptomatic Lumbar Spinal Stenosis," Pain Medicine 13 (2012): 1554-61.

Chapter 9

Back surgery leaves behind a trail of human wreckage: Anthony F. DePalma and Richard H. Rothman, "Surgery of the Lumbar Spine," Clinical Orthopaedics and Related Research 63 (1969): 162-70. Despite their apparent pessimism, both authors went on to distinguished clinical and academic careers within the field.

Japanese study finds generally favorable long-term outcomes for standard discectomy: Etsuro Yorimitsu et al., "Long-Term Outcomes of Standard Discectomy for Lumbar Disc Herniation: A Follow-Up Study of More than 10 Years," Spine 6 (2001): 652-57.

Excellent outcomes with endoscopic discectomy: Xiaotao Wu et al., "Microendoscopic Discectomy for Lumbar Disc Herniation: Surgical Technique and Outcome in 873 Consecutive Cases," Spine 23 (2006): 2689-94.

Excellent outcomes for patients treated with endoscopic transforaminal discectomy: Thomas Hoogland et al., "Endoscopic Transforaminal Discectomy for Recurrent Lumbar Disc Herniation: A Prospective, Cohort Evaluation of 262 Consecutive Cases," Spine 9 (2008): 973-78.

Incidence of complications of endoscopic discectomy fell markedly during the study period: Wu et al., "Microendoscopic Discectomy," 2692-93.

Japanese study found high levels of residual back pain after discectomy: Yorimitsu et al., "Long-Term Outcomes."

About 12.5 percent of discectomy patients had repeat herniation: Yorimitsu et al., "Long-Term Outcomes."

Hoogland found a 4.6 recurrence rate for disc herniation within two years of ETD surgery: Hoogland et al., "Endoscopic Transforaminal Discectomy," 975.

American Pain Society found little evidence for spinal fusion as a treatment for simple discogenic low back pain: Roger Chou et al., "Surgery for Low Back Pain: A Review of the Evidence for an American Pain Society Clinical Practice Guideline," Spine 10 (2009): 1094-109.

Better results for spinal fusion with strict patient selection criteria: Seiji Ohtori et al., "Surgical Versus Nonsurgical Treatment of Selected Patients With Discogenic Low Back Pain: A Small-Sized Randomized Trial," Spine 5 (2011): 347-54.

Spinal fusion moderately superior to nonsurgical treatment in cases of symptomatic spinal stenosis: Chou et. al., "Low Back Pain."

About 27 percent of lumbar spinal surgery patients showed signs of adjacent segment degeneration: Xiao-Peng Xia, Hong-Lin Chen, and Hong-Bin Cheng, "Prevalence of Adjacent Segment Degeneration after Spine Surgery: A Systematic Review and Meta-analysis," Spine Publish Ahead of Print (2012), doi: 10.1097/BRS.0b013e318273a2ea.

Australians achieve good short-term outcomes with CHARITE disc prosthetic: Matthew N. Scott-Young et al., "Clinical and Radiological Mid-Term Outcomes of Lumbar Single-Level Total Disc Replacement," Spine Publish Ahead of Print (2011), doi: 10.1097/BRS.0b013e3182345aa2.

2012 Cochrane Review raises questions about the effectiveness and long-term safety of total disc replacement surgery: Wilco C. H. Jacobs et al., "Total Disc Replacement for Chronic Discogenic Low Back Pain: A Cochrane Review," Spine 1 (2012): 24-36.

Norwegian study finds increased z-joint arthritis after total disc replacement: Christian Hellum et al., "Adjacent Level Degeneration and Facet Arthropathy After Disc Prosthesis Surgery or Rehabilitation in Patients With Chronic Low Back Pain and Degenerative Disc," Spine 25 (2012): 2063-73.

Spinal fusion may be superior to standard conservative care for discogenic pain: Chou et al., "Low Back Pain."

Discectomy provides short-term benefits superior to non-operative treatment: Chou et al., "Low Back Pain."

Relative benefits of microdiscectomy diminish over time,

insignificant at two years: Heikki Osterman et al., "Effectiveness of Microdiscectomy for Lumbar Disc Herniation: A Randomized Controlled Trial With 2 Years of Follow-up," Spine 21 (2006): 2409-14.

Back surgery more likely to lead to significant or complete relief versus conservative care: Adam M. Pearson et al., "SPORT Lumbar Intervertebral Disk Herniation and Back Pain: Does Treatment, Location, or Morphology Matter?" Spine 4 (2008): 428-35.

Discectomy surgery was cost-effective in SPORT subjects: Anna N. A. Tosteson et al., "The Cost Effectiveness of Surgical Versus Nonoperative Treatment for Lumbar Disc Herniation Over Two Years," Spine 19 (2008): 2108-2115. In addition to patient's quality of life, the team considered economic costs such as work-related productivity. In contrast to early studies, the team concluded that economic costs did not significantly impact the cost-effectiveness of discectomy surgery in relation to the SPORT participants.

Surgical treatment superior to conservative treatment in patients with symptomatic spinal stenosis: Chou et al., "Low Back Pain."

Chapter 10

Thirteen percent of discectomy patients have severe residual pain ten years later: Etsuro Yorimitsu et al., "Long-Term Outcomes of Standard Discectomy for Lumbar Disc Herniation," Spine 26 (2001): 652.

Thirteen percent of discectomy patients suffered reherniation within ten years: Yorimitsu et al., "Long Term Outcomes," 656.

Randomized, controlled trial found significant benefits to SCS versus revision surgery: Rod S. Taylor, Jean-Pierre Van Buyten, and Eric Buchser, "Spinal Cord Stimulation for Chronic Back and Leg Pain and Failed Back Surgery Syndrome: A Systematic Review and Analysis of Prognostic Factors," Spine 1 (2004): 152, 154-155.

Systematic review of spinal cord stimulation as a treatment for FBSS: Taylor et al., "Spinal Cord Stimulation," 152-60.

Systematic review finds lead migration in 13.5 percent of SCS patients, breakage in 7.6 percent of patients: Timothy Deer, Jonathan

Carlson, and Patrick W. Hogan, "Neuromodulation for Lumbrosacral Radicular Pain," in iSpine: Evidence-Based Interventional Spine Care, ed. Michael DePalma (New York: Demos Medical Publishing, 2012), 244.

Chapter 11

MRI results not very useful to primary care doctors: John J. You et al., "Patterns of Care After Magnetic Resonance Imaging of the Spine in Primary Care," Spine 1 (2012): 51-59.

Relatively few patients referred for surgical evaluation ultimately have surgery: You et al., "Patterns of Care," 51.

Acute low back pain tends to recur in worsening episodes: Ronald Donelson, Greg McIntosh, and Hamilton Hall, "Is It Time to Rethink the Typical Course of Low Back Pain?" Physical Medicine and Rehabilitation 6 (2012): 394-401. This paper also discusses physicians' misconceptions, including the flawed but oft-cited 1966 paper suggesting a benign course for low back pain.

Letter to the editor of Spine calls for additional research to determine which patients may need early intervention: James F. Wyss, Gregory E. Lutz, and Elizabeth E. LaSalle, "RE: Is It Time to Rethink the Typical Course of Low Back Pain?" Spine 4 (2012): 1024.

Back pain patients with high blood sugar are more disabled one year after diagnosis: Philip Wilkens et al., "Patients With Chronic Low Back Pain and Lumbar Degeneration in Primary Care: A Cohort Study," Spine 1 (2012): 65. While the pattern was statistically significant, it's also worth noting that only twelve of the two hundred fifty participants actually registered high blood sugar at follow-up.

Twin study suggests a little excess weight may protect the spine against degenerative changes: T. Videman et al., "Challenging the Cumulative Injury Model: Positive Effects of Greater Body Mass on Disc Degeneration," Spine 1 (2010): 26-31.

Obese people are more likely to develop chronic low back pain: Ingrid Heuch et al., "Body Mass Index as a Risk Factor for Developing Chronic Low Back Pain," Spine 2 (2013): 133.

Back pain symptoms improved in morbidly obese patients after bariatric surgery: Zvi Lidar et al., "Intervertebral Disc Height Changes after Weight Reduction in Morbid Obese Patients, Its Effect on Life Quality, Radicular and Low Back Pain," Spine 23 (2013): 1947.

ABOUT THE AUTHOR

Ronald M Lieberman, D.O. is nationally recognized expert in the diagnosis and treatment of an array of painful spinal disorders. He is a board-certified physiatrist in both Physical Medicine and Rehabilitation, as well as Pain Management.

Patients seek treatment with Dr. Lieberman who suffer from pain, both acute neck, shoulder and back pain–with or without nerve injuries or sciatica–as well as orthopedic medicine or nerve pain. He pairs proactive patient treatment plans with non-surgical therapies for muscle, tendon and ligament strains and tears as well as stable fractures and arthritis. Trapped nerve syndromes, such as carpal tunnel, and cartilage tears can also be treated with the latest technologies.

His practice offers state-of-the-art techniques and individualized, holistic solutions. His approach encompasses alternative regenerative therapies for conditions that coincide or mimic spine-referred pain such as hip or extremity-referred pain from the back or neck. These conditions may be treated with state-of-the-art ultrasound guided procedures to facilitate individualized treatment modules.

Ronald M Lieberman, D.O. is committed to providing the best possible individualized care. Patients benefit from his ability to quickly diagnose the source of their pain, followed by individually designed treatment plans. Some require only corrective exercises, while therapeutic injection procedures may also be indicated to complete rehabilitation. His goal is to relieve pain and help patients return to the daily activities they enjoy.

His unique range of services, dedicated staff and coordinated expertise, allow Dr. Lieberman to deliver the highest standard of care. He truly puts himself in the shoes of his patients by actively listening to their concerns.

Made in the USA
Monee, IL
12 September 2026

62979098R00105